My lessons on Holistic Health

Dr Arleen De León Robert. PhD.

ISBN: 9798773862963

DEDICATION

First of all, of course, to Him who told me a few years ago that I had not chosen my profession, but that He had chosen it for me. You have always been there even with my qualms and our disagreements in terms over what, how, when and where I should work. I only have to add that You have always been right and I want to thank you for the support and vote of confidence.

"Praise the Lord, my soul, and forget not all his benefits — who forgives all your sins and HEALS ALL YOUR DISEASES, who redeems your life from the pit and crowns you with love and compassion." Psalm 103: 2-4 (New International Version). Thank you my Lord.

CONTENT

ACKNOWLEDGEMENTS

To my family, patients, teachers, colleagues... Thank you for your company on this voyage

INTRODUCTION

We are the sum of our experiences, our beliefs and of the environment in which we were raised. However, our totality is also influenced by the different roles we play throughout life. Among many things, I am a woman, I am a Christian and I am a doctor, and each one of those facets influences the other to mold my views and my actions ahead of the events that God allows me to live.

Being a Christian doctor makes me not only see and treat the biological side of disease, but also compels me to understand that there are other types of illnesses which affect the third sphere and which, either due to apathy or ignorance, we overlook. These are spiritual diseases.

But do not be confused, this book is not an instruction book about medicine. It is a collection of my experiences with the pathologies that affect the body, soul and spirit. In it, I talk about topics like the origin of disease, its development or physiopathology, as well as its treatment from a Christian point of view. In other words, I analyze spiritual experiences from my perspective as a doctor. One facet in my life that influences the other. I also add an extra chapter which includes anecdotes about my education and medical practice.

I firmly believe that the Lord has inspired me to share these autobiographical experiences in my practice so that you can see that faith and science are not incompatible. On the contrary, they are appropriate and desirable. I hope you receive this as a blessing.

With love, Lyly.

HOLISTIC HEALTH

According to the World Health Organization (WHO), the definition of health is: "Health is a state of complete physical, mental and social well-being and not merely the absence of disease or infirmity." Each person is made up of three elements: body, soul and spirit. Each element has its own needs which must be met to feel satisfied. The God-made-man was not an exception. Being in communion with the Spirit, he is taken to a desert where he is challenged in his three spheres. The first, a bodily need, hunger. "If my food does not come from a God-approved origin, I do not want it!"

After seeing his enemy's determination to be honest, he approaches and decides that it is the turn of his intellect and emotions "Dare!" The opponent told him, "live the risk". God will deliver you anyway because you are His child." The adrenaline that began to run through Jesus' veins was stopped by the "No!" that came from his lips, "I only undertake my challenges and adventures if they are approved by Him."

Now a little desperate to find what to accuse Him of, He decides to touch His spiritual area and tries to bribe Him to change His devotion. "Leave that God of poverty and limitations. I and my riches are a better cause for worship. We will give you greatness without so many laws or restrictions." What good is it for me to gain the whole world now, Jesus thought, if in the end my soul will go to eternal perdition with the devil? So he answers, "If I want to be saved, I can only serve and worship God. So go devil, do not bother me any more." (Matthew 4: 1-11).

Jesus came as man, not just to die so that through his sacrifice we could be saved. He also came to show us that it is possible to live in harmony with God, with its benefits for our body, soul and spirit. God bless us.

"The devil set the same traps for Jesus as he sets for us in order to make us sin, except that Jesus never sinned. That is why he can understand how difficult it is for us to obey God. So, when we are in need, let us then approach God's throne of grace with confidence, so that we may receive mercy and find grace to help us in our time of need." Hebrews 4:15-16- NIV.

PHYSIOPATHOLOGY: THE ORIGIN OF DISEASE

There are a few theories among Christians regarding the origin of disease: whether it is always caused by demons, or if only some of them are. Which do I think is true? I will keep my opinion personal. What I can assure you is that illness is an abnormality, an unbalance; something that is altered and is, therefore, susceptible to be normalized, balanced and organized. In other words, the correct situation would be that what is damaged should be mended; with no regard to whether the cause is physical, mental or spiritual.

As an example, I will tell you some of my own experiences:

1-One night I got up and I felt that I could not open my eyes properly. When I looked at myself in the mirror, they looked as if a big, strong, jealous man had taken revenge for my infidelity: they were swollen, bruised and red.

The diagnosis from the specialist was a probable ocular allergy that made my eyes look like that. I took everything: antiallergenics, anti-inflammatories, etc... I used various types of eye drops and... nothing. Weeks went by and I was walking around with big, dark glasses everywhere all the time, until I went on a missionary trip to the province of San Juan de la Manguana, in my country of origin, the Dominican Republic. During prayers, the allergy went as quickly as it came, without my knowing how I had got it, but with a strong suspicion of how I was healed.

2-Oh, those bodily aches and pains! Especially in the back, which would affect me now and then; always curiously associated with the beginning of fasting, a time of penance, or if pray a little longer. I already suspected it, but it was confirmed by the Lord through a preacher that visited my church.

3-Some lesions on my skin, I had to use long sleeves for months even though the temperatures here in Murcia reached more than 40 degrees. I visited dermatologists, I took and applied an infinite number of medicines, all strong. And the lesions? Perfectly well, thank you very much; as if the treatment had nothing to do with them. In the end, I compared myself with Job and said: "Lord: I need double healing and blessings for this mange. I forgot about it and stopped taking medication and they disappeared: without any apparent reason as to why, either for me nor the doctors who saw me.

Well, between the dermatitis of unknown origin and reading a book called "God's Generals" these days, an old query has occurred to me again: whatever the cause of my illness, whether it be an attack of the devil or something natural, it is part of what the Lord wishes for me; as He provided what is necessary for my health on the cross of Calvary. In other words, God's decision has been made, the promise is given, the power is available. So, why don't we perform miracles on ourselves, our brothers and family, and amongst non-believers so they change their minds? Because no matter how much of an atheist you are, if you heal, or see someone you know heal, you will believe, of course, you will.

What is the origin of diseases? I cannot give just one definitive answer to this, as I do not have it; and if someone has the answer, I invite them to give it to me and everyone reading this. What I do know is that the lack of exercising of God's authority is something I have to resolve in my own life.

We are the generation of the last times. Believe it or not, the world has nothing left to give, and we have to comply with our calling on earth, but without power, we will never achieve it. A tepid "Christ loves you", or a noisy sermon, or if we jump up and down speaking tongues, it is not going to impress non-believers. We will only achieve it if the person is healed; if his marriage is mended; if he is freed from problems; if we prophesy and it comes true; or if we tell him about His life, work and miracles through the gift of science.

I wish the purpose of God to be accomplished in me 100%. It is true that I feel intimidated when I leave my comfort zone, as well as the attacks I will receive; but I am going to appropriate a sentence I read from Jim Elliot: "He is no fool who gives what he cannot keep, gaining that which he cannot lose"

"I looked for someone among those who would build up the wall and stand before me in the gap on behalf of the land so I would not have to destroy it, but I found no one." Ezequiel 22:30. Remembering this quote, I dress myself up in courage and I ask the Lord to sign me up to his lines, so that he teach me to take what was already given to me; or believe what already is. Now I ask you to follow me in saying as Isaiah:

"Then I heard the voice of the Lord saying, "Whom shall I send? And who will go for us?" And I said, "Here am I. Send me!" Isaiah 6:8

The fever is not in the bedsheets...

It was when I was studying medicine. Younger and more inexperienced, I was interested in learning everything I could about the target of the fight in my career: disease. That is why, while I was waiting for the doctor in charge of the surgery I was assigned to as a student, I would ask the patients why they had come to the surgery.

The woman was about 65-70 years old. After telling me a long list of aches and pains, she pauses; and looking straight at me she says: "I was born prematurely, you know." She was certain that that would explain the origin of all her ailments. The other patients looked at me doubtfully, looking to me, the aspiring doctor, to confirm this curious theory. I could not to it; and I think I should apologize, because so many years and studies later, I still cannot find the relation between this lady's many aches and pains and her premature birth.

Just like that lady, many of us would have loved a good beginning in something, but it has not been possible. But what is possible, is to not allow a dark past to cast a shadow over the rest of our lives, or our near future. Ask the Lord for strength. Leave the lament behind of what could have been and, with His help, discover and enjoy what is ahead. May the Lord give us wisdom.

"Brothers *and sisters, I do not consider myself yet to have taken hold of it. But one thing I do: Forgetting what is behind and straining toward what is ahead."* Philippians 3:13

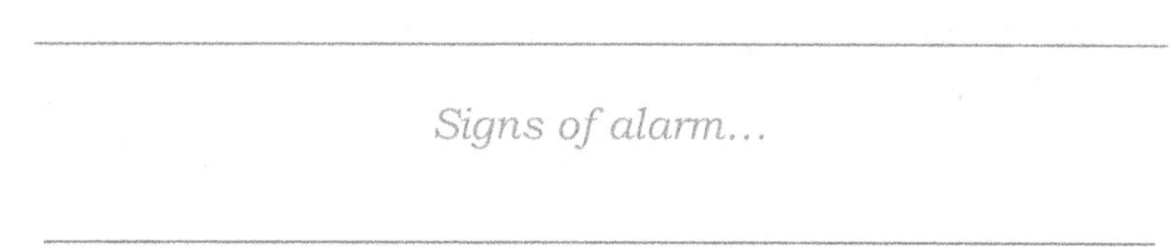

Signs of alarm...

The word "emotion" comes from the Latin "emovere" (move toward); which tells us about the capacity we have to move in a situation (closer or further) influenced by feelings, which are our guide for labelling each situation as favorable or not, and whether we should get closer or further from such a situation depending on how we have classified it.

That is why the Lord allows us to have emotions. Good emotions are totally justified; thanks to them we can do good, feel good and be where we are meant to. But what about the bad ones? Well, we can conclude in accordance with the definition, that these are useful as signs of alarm which tell us to move away from bad situations. For example, if a situation makes me feel anger, regret, fear, envy, etc, then I need to move away from it, and so everything will be solved. But things are not always so black and white, there are other colours and different shades.

Today I want to talk about those situations that should give us good emotions, but that strangely make us feel the opposite. Mary received a certain thing! The correct feelings of the people around Mary should be of happiness because instead of Mary being in a situation of need, she has received a blessing. But on many occasions, that is not how things go. And that doesn't just happen to Mary's friends, it also happens to me (more than I would like to admit), and if you are honest, it happens to you too! Why Lord? How is it possible that after all these years of knowing you, I still battle against carnal emotions? Why does it bother me that Peter has more or better gifts, Joseph gets more calls to preach, Mary obtained the visa, Louis got married first or that Rose always has a clean house without any effort, while I'm working on mine all day, and it always looks like a pigsty?!

Yes, it is true, we all battle with this. From the most devoted to the least. And do you know what? I dare to go further, God knows this and allows it. Yes, He does. He does not only do it so that, as I've said in another reflection, we dominate these feelings, in some situations he goes an extra mile and accomplishes other purposes. How can a negative emotion be of any use? I will tell you.

The parable of the prodigal son leaves a bittersweet taste depending on the point of view. The older son in the story was an accomplished man, but he did not enjoy what was around him. The chaos that arrived with his younger brother, who was welcomed with open arms, gave him an unpleasant, toxic feeling: envy. Thanks to this, the older brother realized what he was missing out on, so he proceeded to complain and his father made him understand that he wasn't receiving because he wasn't asking, since all the wealth of that family had always been at his disposal.

God allows negative emotions to come to our lives so that we realize that we need to change our state, to advance, to ask, to look for more of His presence. All sorts of emotions will always come knocking on our heart. You need to open the door to the good emotions, not the bad ones, those need to be tamed and you also need to reflect on the causes of their appearance. – I should stop going to that place, it is not good for me, I'm always left feeling sad. So-and-so's ministry is growing more than mine; but instead of hating and defaming him, I should look at what I need to improve in my spiritual life, or how I manage it, so that mine also goes well. Luisa's house is cleaner, it must mean I should work more on mine.

God uses negative emotions to stimulate us. God's aim is not for us to feel them and harm ourselves or others; but for us to feel them and in response move in the right direction. May the Lord bless us.

"Now Esau learned that Isaac had blessed Jacob and had sent him to Paddan Aram to take a wife from there, and that when he blessed him he commanded him, "Do not marry a Canaanite woman," and that Jacob had obeyed his father and mother and had gone to Paddan Aram. Esau then realized how displeasing the Canaanite women were to his father Isaac; so he went to Ishmael and married Mahalath, the sister of Nebaioth and daughter of Ishmael son of Abraham, in addition to the wives he already had." Genesis 28:6-9

Abused...

I was surprised when I heard, I could not believe it. She was known as a strong woman, resolute, an example of how not to put up with anyone's abuse. I was horrified when I heard from her own voice how she had been abused and isolated from her family and friends by some who had promised to love and respect her forever.

What was terrible was that not only did she surprise all

who were listening, it was also a surprise for her. She used to see herself as a woman that would not be dominated, so she was horrified at the thought of having fallen into that sad situation.

Uniting with others (romantically, in friendship, socially, etc.) makes us adopt some of their characteristics, but it also makes us act to adapt ourselves to them. That is also true on a spiritual level.

People that are influenced by abusive spirits generally get married to or relate with people that have already been influenced by abuse and have experienced it in their childhood or youth through the actions of family members or people close to the family. But they meet people that had never previously been influenced (like the girl in the story) but who acquire these influences by relating with them.

Let us pray for the children that are born to homes where one of the parents has evil influences. Let us pray for those who are or have been abused, only the Lord can cut through the grip between the abused soul and the conduct of the abuser, both demonic influences.

And you, who observe all these abnormal conducts in your friends, partner, colleagues... run away as soon as you can. No, it is not true; you will not be able to manage it and you will not make them change. Only God can change people.

"Do not be misled: "Bad company corrupts good character." 1 Corinthians 15:33 (NIVUK)

PHYSICAL PATHOLOGIES

Symptoms of alarm...

Not everything is joy. There is not always delight, I will not lie to you. What I can assure you is that after so many years, I know where to go to if I start having a crisis and that perennial refuge, where I always find solace and answers, never runs out of resources to bring me back my lost peace and joy.

The sadness and the reason for writing, comes after thinking about the people I see every day at work. False physical illnesses that hide an emotional origin or, actual physical illnesses that are conditioned and worsened by psychological elements. I know which medicine cures me, but what do the patients do? How do they battle daily without running for shelter under the love, the power, the mercy of the eternal Lord, their Creator?

He is unique. There are no pills, therapy or advise from professionals; who do not even know how to resolve their own lives, not to mention anyone else's.

Looking at real life I realize that I am enormously privileged. My duty towards myself, and yours towards yourself (we will talk later about our duty to others), is not to move away from the key to true happiness. There is nothing to look for out there.

"And, "If it is hard for the righteous to be saved, what will become of the ungodly and the sinner?" 1 Peter 4:18 (NIV)

Signs of alarm...

The increase in body temperature to above 38° Celsius is defined as a fever. What most people do not know is that the fever itself is not a problem. On the contrary, it is one of the weapons that the Creator gave the body for it to defend itself. How many bacteria, viruses which have passed through our body, have been literally "fried", destroyed by this increase in temperature; without us even noticing their presence? And thanks to the fever this was possible.

Due to ignorance many see it as an enemy. It is true that you should not let it rise too much, but you do not have to rush to get rid of it, especially before it goes up to the debatable 37.5°C mark. If you do, not only are you disabling its effectiveness, but also we do not know if what we are giving it as an "antidote" could cause more harm than the bug itself, which the fever is defending us from.

The same happens in life. There are people that are placed by God to take care of us and to foresee that whatever is approaching will do us harm and they want to protect us. Advice, warnings, limitations, prohibitions... are the rise in temperature that they use to call our attention to something apparently harmless, or insignificant or even pleasant.

I know that the current trend is to reaffirm our freedom of choice but, why don't you affirm your true independence using your intellect to decide whether the person giving you advice is right or not, rather than rush to lower your temperature which will probably help you to avoid a scare in the future? The fever is not in the bedsheets; but what is wrong is not the fever either.

"Ezequiel, I have made you a watchman for the people of Israel; so hear the word I speak and give them warning from me. When I say to a wicked person, 'You will surely die,' and you do not warn them or speak out to dissuade them from their evil ways in order to save their life, that wicked person will die for their sin, and I will hold you accountable for their blood. But if you do warn the wicked person and they do not turn from their wickedness or from their evil ways, they will die for their sin; but you will have saved yourself." Ezekiel 3:17-19

Overload...

Not sleeping, or not sleeping well, is fattening, it sours our character, raises the blood pressure, makes us ill, age earlier... All of this, though said in a simple way, is backed by multiple and reliable scientific investigations.

God ordered the Israelites to rest on Saturday, not to honor the day itself, but to force them to rest as he knew that, be it for greed or obsession, they would force themselves and others to work seven days a week, which would destroy their body, mind and family relationships.

If it is possible, when you have a chance: rest and sleep well; it is not worth the struggling and pushing yourself a little more in detriment to your life. God created you to be a balanced being.

"What do people get for all the toil and anxious striving with which they labor under the sun? All their days their work is grief and pain; even at night their minds do not rest. This too is meaningless." Eclesiastes 2:22-23

"Then he said to them, "The Sabbath was made for man, not man for the Sabbath." Mark 2:27 (NIV)

PATHOLOGIES OF THE SOUL

Alternative medicine

Those things that cannot be seen are also important. We tend to disregard them because they do not stain our clothes, they do not make us run, they do not need any medicine that we can pay for. They are the wounds to the soul. A bad gesture, a bad word… or on the contrary: absence of gestures, absence of words. The bottom line is that the skin of our soul cracks, in some cases even bleeds, with that clear blood that comes out of those modified veins we call eyes.

Do you know what the saddest thing is? We tend to ignore them, we don't talk about them, unaware that it is the first step in healing: acknowledging that you are hurt, that your soul hurts, that it bleeds when you are alone and no one can see you.

Wounds to the soul can also become chronic, we call that the root of bitterness. It can increase so much that it can cripple you, we call that trauma. They can also make us wish to die, as with depression, or wish someone else would die, as with hate.

As you will see, invisible injuries also need healing. There is no pill in the chemist that works miracles, so stop trying. Let us acknowledge that they are there, that they hurt, that they make us bleed in solitude and let us seek health.

If you do not have the means to acquire this eternal remedy for pain, which is forgiveness, look for that Someone that has all the resources to help you acquire it and apply it, Jesus.

"The Spirit of the Lord is on me, because he has anointed me to

proclaim good news to the poor. He has sent me to proclaim freedom for the prisoners and recovery of sight for the blind, to set the oppressed free," Luke 4:18

Peeping its head out, as yet unnamed, there was an emotional pain that nowadays is widely known and suffered: depression.

Sadness, hopelessness, insomnia, grievance, indifference to the gestures we receive from others to cheer us up, etc. David suffered from it and you can see it perfectly described in the Psalm 77. However, noticing the persistence of this anguish, he understands that it is not a problem of external origin (caused by someone else or the environment) so he declares: *"It is my grief"* (v.10)

The Creator was alluding to His trinity when He formed His special creation as a tripartite being. Not only do our body gets ill, our soul and our spirit can as well. David understood it in this way and for his soul's illness he applied a soul's cure *"I will remember the deeds of the Lord; yes, I will remember your miracles of long ago. I will consider all your works and meditate on all your mighty deeds." (vv 10b-12)*

Remember the wonders the Lord did with you; write them down, meditate, reflect and talk to others. Thank the Lord, you are worth it, you are loved, protected, valued, you have a future... If God was with you in the past, he will continue to be in the future. Remember, declare it and be healed of that depression. In the name of Jesus!

"Sacrifice thank offerings to God, fulfill your vows to the

Most High, and CALL ON ME IN THE DAY OF TROUBLE; I will deliver you, and you will honor me." Psalm 50:14-15

Stress...

Stress, anxiety, can come to our lives in two very different ways. One of them is through our feelings and emotions; as when our heart enters a state of unease because of what we feel, be it justified or not. We start the day off badly, our health is weakened, our hormonal and/or enzymatic cycle is altered... All of that can make us feel that we are in crisis.

The other cause is our analytical mind. Here the brain processes real information that lead us to the logical conclusion that the situation is not in our favour, and so we need to do something quickly or we will fail; or that no matter what we do, we are lost.

The origin of the feeling of hopelessness and ruin is not important, Philipians 4: 6,7 tells us that the problem has a real and effective solution:

"Do not be anxious about ANYTHING, but in every situation, by prayer and petition with thanksgiving, present your requests (problems, worries) *to God. And the PEACE OF GOD, which transcends all understanding, will guard your hearts and your minds in Christ Jesus."* The way you got to that hole is not important, look to God. He will rescue you.

<hr>

Autolytic attempt

<hr>

At that moment we were transferring a patient to the hospital, so we were outside when we received the alert: someone had gone to the health centre where I worked to announce they were going to commit suicide, giving the details of where and how.

As we were the only team available and we were very far away, we alerted the coordination centre about the need to take measures to locate the patient and contain him till our arrival. The police force found him in the place he had said earlier and in an attitude of waiting patiently, as on many other occasions. He only threatened suicide so someone would go and find him and so pressurize his family in order to achieve the goal he had set that day (an autolytic gesture).

Manipulations and cries for attention aside, in the life of any human being some situations cannot always be foreseen, they emerge bit by bit, giving off alarm signals, and indicating that, if the measures are not taken they will reach a point of no return, missing the chance to be saved.

To keep quiet, to look the other way acting as though nothing is going on, will only accelerate the tragic ending and will prevent the chance of rescue. Speak, ask for help, try to explain... don't lock yourself up in your limitations or loneliness, maybe it is true that there is nothing you can do, but if you sound the alarm bell and ask for help someone will show up. Start by talking and asking the all-powerful Lord for help. He will make someone appear to help you and listen to you. May the Lord guide you and bless you.

"In my distress I called to the Lord; I cried to my God for help. From his temple he heard my voice; my cry came before

him, into his ears." Psalm 18:6 (New International Version)

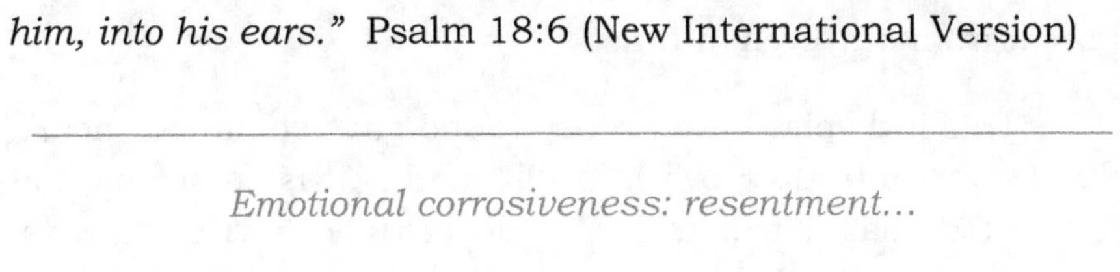

Emotional corrosiveness: resentment...

A visiting preacher, during his ministry in our church, mentioned Ahitofel, David's advisor. He gave a reason for his suicide that is not quite true.

Hidden in the web of time, and if we stay on the surface, we will accept and validate that he commited suicide in a moment of rage and hurt pride, for his advice had not been listened to by Absalom, on how to defeat David. After all, he was considered the best advisor in the kingdom, his advice was taken as a word from God as it was so pertinent and wise.

"Now in those days the advice Ahithophel gave was like that of one who enquires of God. That was how both David and Absalom regarded all of Ahithophel's advice." 2 Samuel 16:23

But if we cleared the spiderweb, what would we find? We would see that many years earlier (I wouldn't be able to say how many) Ahitophel had a son called Eliam (2 Samuel 23:34) and many years later he in turn had a daughter called... Bathsheba (2 Samuel 11:3)

Working together, enjoying the victories given my God, contributing to those victories with your advice or in other ways, but in the end find yourself betrayed... that was something Ahithophel could not get over. Years went by (some writers say eleven) until a chance appeared for Ahithophel to wreak revenge, and he took it.

We can hide from the rest of the world that we hold resentment toward someone, but two people will not miss this detail: God, who knows our hearts, and the enemy who sows the seed that will turn into a plant of bitterness if we do not get rid of it from our lives in time.

This little plant, which has found good soil in our heart, is going to continue growing until the day it is so strong and well-rooted that it will make us do terrible, horrible things, things that had never before crossed our minds. I think that Ahithophel was really a friend of David's, and that his initial intentions for his friendship with the king were for life, but the offense he suffered, with his family becoming an object of scandal, his granddaughter taken, her husband killed by a man that had served, protected, loved and esteemed him, this was something he had to take vengeance for... or not?

David commited a sin and was never going to be held as innocent in the eyes of God. He had to pay for his mistakes with all the misfortune of his family. In many cases the mistakes of others reach us, and affect us too. It is sad and painful but we must strengthen ourselves in the Lord and leave revenge to Him, and not take matters into our own hands.

The mocked friendship of Ahithophel was also avenged by the Lord, for God there are no more beautiful children. If someone has harmed us they will have to meet up with God and give an account of themselves sooner or later. If it seems longer than we would like, we should still rest in Him and let God clean our hearts of all resentment and bitterness, trusting that in the end there will be justice. If Ahithophel had done this instead of allying with David's enemies his life would not have ended so sadly, taking his life due to the fear of punishment for his treason when his old friend returned to the throne.

Let us see, we have overcome the idea of wreaking revenge with our own hands. We have see God work and demand payment from the offender. Is it alright for me to tell people that what happened to brother so-and-so was the Lord exacting payment for what he did to me? The correct answer is: *"Do not gloat when your enemy falls; when they stumble, do not let your heart rejoice, or the Lord will see and disapprove and turn his wrath away from them."* Proverbs 24:17-18

It is not an easy thing to do, I agree with you, being offended and then forgiving; leaving things to the Lord so our thirst for justice is quenched. No, it is not something we can do alone, we need His help; and on occasions, more than once. But what is true, is that it is indispensible for our spiritual health. May God help us not to be resentful.

Therapy in stages...

To arrive somewhere, sometimes we need to go through more than one door. For God to work within a broken relationship, whatever the type, there are times where we have to take the first step, open the first door. Show yourself to be receptive, apologize, speak kindly, smile as you pass... And ask God to open the second door that is always the hardest: heal the wounds and restore lost trust.

"If it is possible, as far as it depends on you, live at peace with everyone." Roman 12:18

Rehabilitating treatment...

I love you, my love...

Those beautiful words are the ones I hear from my mother every time she calls me, between two and four times in each call. What is so special about them? it is that before I never heard her say them; not only had I not heard them in the past from her, but from no one in my close family.

To be honest, there had been many moments when I thought they did not love me; but my relationship with God made me understand that they did, it was just that because of their upbringing, physical and verbal displays of affection were practically non-existent; as I said once before, "no one can give what they do not have".

The natural history of my family relations was interrupted when I moved away from my country. I joined up with another three girls to rent a house while we prepared for our specialization exam. Of the three, I must mention now that I'm on the topic, Nacha, who shared an apartment with me for several years.

I was surprised to hear her talk to her family. I heard her say: I love you, dear, lovely brother or sister, etc... and it struck me as something shocking and strange. And when I heard her refer to them as little short of perfect (and that little bit that was lacking God was making up), it made me feel jealous, and at the same time, made me ask myself bitterly why my family and I could not treat each other that way.

But the change came through me. Nacha does not know how instructive and impacting those words of love she would say to me back then. I never knew how to answer when at the end of a conversation she would say goodbye saying: I love you loads, sis! Or, you're so good! I felt so uncomfortable; so I would say: "Don't say that to me in front of people, they'll think we're weird." Until I started to accept her love and answer back: "I love you loads too."

With my heart in my mouth I started the experiment. I started with my mother and noticed her initial surprise. To be honest I do not know what it felt like to her at the beginning, maybe she thought it was an attack of nostalgia because of the distance between us at that time, but the fact is that I continued to say things to her, while laughing and with a bit of melancholy, in June as in January, whether we were closer or further away. To my father, to my siblings... I talk to everyone of them and tell them I love them, how thankful I am for having them, and I try to erase my tendency to criticize. I try not to point out what we do not have, and point out what we have received from God, receiving from them a similar response.

It is hard to break bad habits, but it is not imposible: *"for the Spirit will help us in our weaknesses"*. Talking between ourselves, the Lord has stated that when speaking we assert that we have not yet achieved something ... it will happen later on. What we do not have... will be supplied by the Lord. No judgement or comparisons. God is with us, and everything will turn out well.

Tell your family you love them, bless them when you talk to them, it is not a mere formality. Sometimes we assume so many things, we think that others "know it" without understanding the profound abyss that could be forming between us. The worst thing is that something can happen and you are not able to tell them.

Try it, at the beginning you will feel fake or forced, but at the end you will realize how important it is to reaffirm family ties and demonstrate your love. So start doing it now.

"Your beginnings will seem humble, so prosperous will your future be." Job 8:7

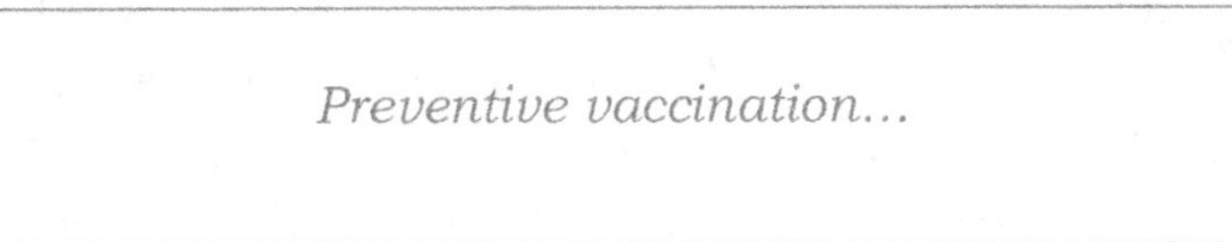

Preventive vaccination...

Someone close that door! Mental oppressions can come to our lives in various forms and for different lengths of time. Some come to minds that are already affected or weakened, but those who do not have previous problems, or who consider themselves to be strong at first, do not escape either. What is more, even the minds of believers are not immune from those savage and destructive attacks to our thoughts and feelings.

In my own experience I see how from a state of tranquillity or even joy, I can go to the most absolute desperation when those malignant thoughts come to visit without warning. Feelings of abandonment, low self-esteem, death wishes ... they arrive at my door with the desire to take up residence in my life. I try to close my door and stop them from entering. I cannot on my own. How do I get rid of those voices without pills, alcohol, psychoanalysis, drugs, without taking my life, without...? Asking Jesus to close the door. He does, and he does so better than any human method.

"And the peace of God, which transcends all understanding, will guard your hearts and your minds in Christ Jesus." Philipians 4:7

You do not have to let them invade you and live in your life. Ask the Lord to close that door.

Opportunistic pathogens...

It is foul play when someone sees you are going through a bad patch and takes advantage by entering your house and staying there without being wanted or invited. I do not know if this happens much in one's natural life, but it always happens in spiritual life. Many call it trauma when the event was violent, others may say "I'm a bit sensitive after that", without understanding that a new guest is living in their lives.

Depression after losses; fear and/or anxiety after a scare: the lack of self-esteem after someone rejects you... It is very true that we were created with emotions, which were given to us so we could react to potential danger or relieve our feelings about something painful; but what is not normal is that we live all our lives as slaves of those negative feelings that limit us.

Cry if you have lost someone. Make a move if you need to resolve something. Protect yourself if something threatens you but give your anxiety an expiry date, do not allow it to live with you. Whether it be it a big or small problem, it is over. You need to keep on living, there will be more than enough time to die.

"Whatever your hand finds to do, do it with all your might, for in the realm of the dead, where you are going, there is neither working nor planning nor knowledge nor wisdom." Ecclesiastes 9:10

Remember: your Creator made you so you could live the years He has given you in the best possible way and His son Jesus Christ came to earth so that through Him you will move away from sin and live plentifully. He does not want "what happened" to determine "what happens" or "what will happen" in your life. Kick out those invaders! Only you and God can live in your house.

"The thief comes only to steal and kill and destroy; I have come that they may have life, and have it to the full." John 10:10 (NIV)

Acquired immunodeficiencies...

Spectacular and sad at the same time; there is no other way of defining the feeling that invaded me when I learned the results. Sad, for how close to home it was; she was more than a cousin, she was like an older sister. I detected with just one glance a small mass in a place that it should not be.

Spectacular, because I could prove, even though I was just a medical student, how all the blood cells taken by the same laboratory decreased in size suddenly after one week without bleeding or other intervention that would justify it. The only visible cause, the depression my cousin fell into after learning that the pathological anatomy determined that the mass on her neck was from malignant origin.

Without strength, some say to me; nothing brings me joy, say others; I lack creativity, little things annoy me, I am indifferent to gestures of affection... These and other comments I have heard in my surgery, speaking to siblings, family, friends and even I probably said them on some occasions. What we do not realize sometimes or do not take into consideration, is that sadness does not only affect emotions, it also affects your physical health.

Diseases get worse when our emotional state is low, when we stop fighting. Have you ever noticed that patients with cancer which has been evolving for years and detected by accident, die faster when they find out what they have? Before, they did not even feel discomfort, until they were diagnosed by chance. God's wise words warn us: *"The human spirit can endure in sickness, but a crushed spirit who can bear?"* Proverbs 18:14

God made humans able to battle till the last moment. Our spirit does not only keep us standing, it also limits the damage of sickness and makes the results of the treatment better. Cheer up, and cheer the person that needs it. And if you cannot do it alone; do what I do, I take refuge in the one who always brings joy to the heart: God (oh and he also brings health) May the Lord bless us!

PATHOLOGIES OF THE SPIRIT

Correct nutritional deficiencies...

I saw her hesitate before asking the question, "Can I give my baby water?" and to clarify she continued, "And how will I know that she's thirsty?" My answer was the same as any other paediatrician: "Don't worry, breast milk has all the nutrients and water that newborns need. When they feel a need, they ask for the breast, whether it is hunger, thirst or even affection and comforting. The mother's breast is the answer to all your problems." Like God, I nearly told her.

I know, it sounds a bit strange, but I couldn't help the comparison. We spend large portions of our lives looking for formulas that are mere imitations of the essential and unique milk that has all we need because it was designed for that. Men and women were made to depend on their Creator and to languish and feel frustrated, incomplete and anaemic if they do not have their original spiritual food.

God provides material, and also spiritual things; even comfort and the satisfaction to enjoy both. Do you feel empty even with everything you have? Do you feel "hungry" even with everything you have? Leave the "substitutes" and feed yourself with the "real" stuff. Get closer to your Creator.

"On the last and greatest day of the festival, Jesus stood and said in a loud voice, "Let anyone who is thirsty come to me and drink. Whoever believes in me, as Scripture has said, rivers of living water will flow from within them." John 7:37-38. (NIV)

Abandon spiritual sedentariness...

Through my profession I know first-hand how beneficial exercise is for your health, and I highly recommend it. But not just for physical health. To people that complain about stress I also recommend an activity as a means of entertainment and relaxation.

I must confess something: I do not like it. I do not understand people that go to the gym injured so as to not miss a class. – When you get used to it... they tell me, but I've been going almost uninterruptedly, and it seems, the famous endorphins (satisfaction hormones) produced after exercise have no effect on me. So, Lyly, perhaps you do it because you know the benefit it gives in the long term? Don´t judge me so well, the only thing that motivates me to "move myself" faster is when I see how quickly the my accumulated fat moves.

Equally, not everyone likes spiritual exercises. We love God and we wish for a healthy relationship with him; but in order to pray, fast, reading the word, etc. in a disciplined manner, you need a lot of will power that not everyone has; and many times find themselves, as I do, with a threat to their stability to do spiritual exercises, which, although they do not enjoy them, are key to maintaining devotional health, now and in the future. Do you wish to stop feeling the weight of your sins? Exercise!

"Therefore, since we are surrounded by such a great cloud of witnesses, let us throw off everything that hinders and the sin that so easily entangles. And let us run with perseverance the race marked out for us," Hebrews 12:1 (NIV)

Ask for a doctor's appointment...

He had a problem; bigger, smaller, different from ours ... but it was his problem. He decides to tell God about it in prayer, in the middle of which he pauses and reminds him: *"You are my God; LORD, hear my prayers"* (Psalm 140: 6b). We should always do as David did, not because of God, because He does not forget, but because of ourselves.

Do I have a problem with my health? with my family? with finances? at work? ... What should I do, complain? Go from one place to another? Allow myself to die? No, I must remind myself: I am not alone or helpless, I have a God. I will cry out to Him until he hears the voice of my prayers.

Many times we are only a prayer of faith away from our response. I know that in the midst of the pressure of the problem it is difficult for us to find faith in our doubts, but let us be advised by David, who in the same Psalm reinforces his faith by remembering what God did for him in the past (v.7); asking for what he needs in his present (v.8); dreaming about what he expects God to do in the future (vv.9-11); declaring God's faithfulness (v.12) and giving thanks because he trust that He will hear him (v.13). Remember that you have a God. He is waiting to hear you.

"But I have put my hope in the Lord; I hope in the God of my salvation. My God will listen to me!" Micah 7: 7.

Do not abuse your body...

The truth is that they look like lanterns, or rather, lanterns look like them. I am talking about eyes. Jesus already called them a lamp in the Gospels, and it is to be expected, since through them vision is produced: our inner being captures what happens on the outside.

But here comes the curious thing, Jesus not only points out its vital and obvious function, but also highlights a more spiritual one: - *The eye is the lamp of the body* (Luke 11:34) ... because it not only captures what happens outside; they also reflect it inward, influencing what happens within. That is why we must ask ourselves: How do we see things that happen? What is our attitude, what are our intentions? Do we look with malice, with pride, with greed? Do we look at the lives of others to criticize, to wish bad things to happen to them; I rush to see how someone with whom I have had problems falls? Or do I look with kindness, with innocence, with mercy?

The important thing about this, according to what the Lord tells us, is that depending on the light or darkness with which I look, my body will receive it back. Anxiety, depression, bitterness, perversions, physical illnesses ... stop looking in a way that you should not, or see what you should not, if you want to be liberated.

"The lamp of the body is the eye; when your eye is good, your whole body is also full of light; but when your eye is evil, your body is also in darkness" Matthew 6:22

Obey medical orders...

Jonah was very hurt by the people of Nineveh. He had heard and seen how they had mistreated his people for years; so he was not very happy that God sent him as a prophet to that country to warn its inhabitants that if they did not convert from their wickedness they would be destroyed (Jonah 3: 4).

He knew God, he knew that if the Ninevites decided to repent (as indeed happened), God was so good and merciful that He would surely forgive them. *"And God saw what they did, that they turned from their evil way; and He repented of the evil that He had said he would do to them, and he did not do it."* Jonah 3:10.

The forgiveness of offences has two sides: 1- The one that must be granted by the aggrieved person and 2- The one that corresponds to God. If we understand that it is our duty to forgive, both because it is an important requirement for ourselves to be able to heal, and because God asks us to; We must bear in mind that this forgiveness must be complete: we cannot get angry if we see that the other person is not doing badly in life, nor that the bad that we have sometimes wished him or her is happening to him. Allow forgiveness to be complete.

"Jonah did not like at all that God saved the city and was enraged. Then he prayed to the Lord and said: Lord, was not this what I said when I was in my own country? That was why at first I tried to flee to Tarsis. I knew that you are a good God, that you show great compassion, you do not get angry easily, you are full of love and you are willing to change your plans for punishment." Jonah 4: 1-2 (NIV)

Trust your doctor, He knows what He is doing...

It was incomprehensible to him. He was sitting there, bathed, dressed, calmly paying attention; but people continued to be afraid of him. Before it had been foreseeable: dirty, naked, hurting himself and others; screaming, walking among graves ... but now?

As I listened to him, I marveled in the opposite way from the Gadarene in Luke 8: 37-9. -I had not suffered from blood pressure before; I was told, when they monitored it, it was always fine, but since that event (fright, death of a relative, argument, etc ...) I have to take pills and sometimes it becomes difficult to control. He was not lying to me, at that time it was quite high. Hence my question: Why does it not surprise us when we show signs of a physical disease without a biological cause or a prior pathophysiological change? And why do we doubt or reject it when God liberates or wants to liberate us (through healing, cleansing, providing ...) or someone else? Is it acceptable for something (yes, something) to take possession of an area of our life permanently in order to harm us, and not for God to perform a miracle? Let us review our faith to see whose side it is on. It is very likely that seeking, accepting and celebrating God's work at that moment of need is all the solution you need.

"He (Jesus) could not do any miracles there, except lay his hands on a few sick people and heal them. He was amazed at their lack of faith. Then Jesus went around teaching from village to village" Mark 6: 5-6.

Do not hide any symptoms

"There was a time when I refused to acknowledge how sinful I was. But I was weak and miserable and I groaned all day. Day and night his (God's) hand weighed on me. My strength evaporated like water on a sunny day." Psalm 32: 3-4.

"God knows everything" it is true, but in His justice He asks you to recognize your fault and ask for forgiveness (from Him ... and if there is someone else affected, too) for the wrong you have done.

David, confident of God's love, fell silent after his sin, forgetting that in addition to being loving, God is just, and so he had to suffer the consequences of his wandering. Physical illness, anxiety, depression, family tragedies, professional failures ... are part of the consequences that David brought upon himself and that we can carry when we persist in what we know is wrong. Let us evaluate our behavior, ask for forgiveness, and turn away from error. God will be happy to restore us.

"Then I acknowledged my sin to you and did not cover up my iniquity.
I said, "I will confess my transgressions to the LORD*." And you forgave the guilt of my sin".* Psalm 32: 5 (NIV)

Do not forget to take the doses of medication

Although in recent reflections we have spoken of leaving the past behind in order to extend ourselves to the future, I must correct myself, since this is not absolutely true. There are times when we will have to turn to the past if we want to stand firm in the present and victoriously achieve a future. An example of this was Joseph.

After the injustices, abuses and lies to which he was subjected, he thanked God for allowing him to forget so much misfortune; since this not only opened the way for him to receive his blessing, it also allowed him to enjoy it: two things, dear brothers and sisters, that do not always go together.

However, although the key for Joseph to be able to enjoy the future was to forget the bad things of the past, to remain standing in a present full of tragedies until he obtained what was promised, the key was to remember. Yes, in remembering what God had told him when he was still a young man who had not yet been battered by life.

If you have already passed through this process or if you have already received the blessing, forget what happened. But if the test is still your present, remember again and again that promise that God gave you in the past, it will keep you standing until you arrive safely in your future.

"Seek strength in the LORD, always turn to His help. Remember his signs and wonders and the righteous decisions that he has uttered." Psalm 105: 4-5 *(NIV)*

Follow the treatment, it is what will make you feel better

Oppression. Any thought or feeling that brings you restlessness, anguish, sadness, a sense of disability or divine helplessness, does not come from God, it does not come from you, it is an oppression. You can seek help in things, and even other people can offer it to you with all the best intention, but they will not be able to break the bonds. Only what comes covered or supported by the anointing of the Saint is what will be able to liberate you.

Do not feel useless, do not feel like a hopeless sinner. You have a God who knows that you do not want to be like this, and since you belong to Him, He wants you to be free. Seek His help, let Him work. Your chains will be broken.

"The peace of God will guard all your thoughts and feelings because you belong to Jesus Christ. His peace can do much better than our human mind." Philippians 4: 7

How long will the treatment last? Until the wound heals

A patient complained to me about the nurse who had treated him. Apparently she had a bad attitude. "When she treats me, she always rubs the wound so much that it ends up bleeding again." I congratulated him, "You have an excellent nurse." "What do you mean?!" he answered in surprise. Then I explained to him, "When she rubs, she removes the dead tissue out of the way and searches until she finds the tissue where there are blood vessels (that's why it bleeds); because it is through them that the elements capable of regenerating new tissue emerge."

There will always be things that we must FORGET if we want to heal and keep moving forward. A wound will never close if it has any putrefaction inside. The dead tissue must be removed from the middle and so, only then, will the new tissue appear. Instead, there will be things that we must preserve if we want the wound to heal and new tissue to grow.

We each have our spiritual strengths. I think of myself (and I hope) that I am a person who believes what God tells her, no matter how hard it is to believe: if He spoke it, it will happen. My problem comes when I forget what He has already told me. For this reason, I always make an effort to write it down so that I can remember it from time to time.

Today the heavenly doctor advises us that everything that prevents us from moving forward must be removed, left behind, forgotten; and instead, we must strive to STUDY, REMEMBER, and PUT INTO PRACTICE His word, which is what gives us life.

"Never stop reading the book of the Law; study it day and night, and put it into practice, so that you will be successful in everything you do." Joshua 1: 8

Attend your medical check-ups: Will I have faith?

For my dear sister E., because through your question God has given me an answer.

Having faith is a condition that leads you to obedient action, even though you do not see a logical reason or do not get an expected ending. This has been important for me to understand, because when I lose sight of what it is to have faith, I reach a state of frustration and discouragement, like the one I was going through until recently.

I just came to understand it recently, while talking to a dear sister after a women's gathering. She told me that lately she did not feel capable of having the faith that many preachers speak of, when they achieve everything they want just by "decree" and that she would like to have Abraham's faith because of a personal situation she was going through. However, seeing that the years go by and that this has not been resolved, she feels that her faith is not of sufficient quality.

I assure you that I was not the one who answered her, since the information had not reached my brain correctly when I heard the following words come out of my mouth: "But your faith does resemble that of Abraham. You have sacrificed having those situations in your home under control in order to follow Christ. You have put up with not having them resolved as many people promise, and yet you have decided to remain faithful, because you believe in God: that is having faith.

Abraham obeyed despite the fact that the order seemed to be for no reason. He had been faithful to God and had waited for that blessing for years, so it must have seemed like a real injustice to go through that situation after so many trials, but even so, he continued to obey.

We should understand that he did not know that in the end Isaac was going to be freed from death. He really thought that he was going to die. We can read this later in Hebrews 11:17. There it tells us that he obeyed and was going to give him up as a sacrifice because he trusted that if God allowed Isaac to die, it was because God was going to resurrect him, since God had promised to give him descendants through him. So he carried on obeying: that is faith.

Yes, that is faith, but it is also faith when, without having promises from God that something will end well, without having the hope of a miracle, we continue to obey and love God.

Please do not misunderstand me, I believe in a God of miracles. The acts of God in my favor have been many and marvelous. I have seen him perform miracles in my life when everyone said it was impossible. I have seen Him provide for me in the midst of absolute scarcity, heal me, set me free, give me comfort in the midst of sadness, guard me and protect me from open and hidden dangers. He has revealed hidden things to me and has shown me in advance situations that I would go through later.

I believe everything of God, because I have seen Him do everything. But I admit that at some point I have forgotten that He is sovereign; and I have started to get upset because I forget that faith is not forcing Him to do what I want, but to trust that I will see what HE HAS TOLD ME TO DO, AND IN THE TIME THAT HE DECIDES TO DO IT. So what if He decides not to answer that request, or not to answer it in the time that I hope He does, I must continue to believe in Him and obey Him: that is faith.

In recent years, Christianity has gone from a doctrine of suffering everything, without the slightest right to anything, thinking that obtaining a blessing was a sin, to not wanting to suffer the slightest annoyance or difficulty, since that means that if we have problems, we are in sin! and all this in the name of faith. But the same Bible that says: "*Every good gift and every perfect gift comes ... from the Father of lights.*" It is the same that says: "*In the world you will have affliction ...*" True faith leads us to love him, follow him, and serve him in both James 1:17 and John 16:33.

May the Lord help us to trust Him and follow Him whatever our situation is, that is faith.

"*Shadrach, Meshach and Abednego answered him: "Your Majesty, that is not something that worries us. If the God we worship wants it that way, he is able to free us from the fire and the power of His Majesty. But even if he does not want to. to do so, we do not intend to worship that golden statue."* Daniel 3: 16-18 (NIV).

HEALTH AND HEALTHCARE IN TIMES OF ANY PANDEMIC

Immunization

Day after day she was describing a new symptom to me while playing down its importance, which nevertheless struck me as typical. Fever, general discomfort, tiredness, lack of appetite ... "You should get tested." I recommended. "I don't have that virus" she answered in her usual energetic way, to the point where my suspicion turned to alarm when I found after repeating my advice to her over a period of a few days, that she no longer answered back. "I'm already much better" she insisted on the phone in order to calm me down.

However, the truth was suddenly revealed. When walking down the street she fainted and had to be helped by a passersby and then taken to the emergency room. What to do when you can do nothing, either because you are far away, because there are no resources or because there is simply no solution? Well, when you need a miracle, the only thing you can do is go to the only One who can do miracles and ask Him. The answer came even before the diagnosis: "Tell my daughter that this disease is not for death. He still has a purpose to fulfill". Water in the middle of the desert. The result of the test no longer mattered; God had answered us through an unknown prophet. Three days later, the test result: positive for COVID19 and tomography revealing secondary pneumonia.

"I didn't want to worry them, but I thought I was dying" my mother later confessed to me.

Our lives are in God's hands. We depart when He decides. But our main victory does not lie in our staying longer on this earth; but in the fact that He is with us, wherever we are. Have you made your peace with God?

If we live, we live for the Lord; and if we die, we die for the Lord. So, whether we live or die, we belong to the Lord. For this very reason, Christ died and returned to life so that he might be the Lord of both the dead and the living. Romans 14: 8-9

Immunity support...

"It happened one month before he looked so seriously ill that we all thought that he would not be saved. That thought repeatedly came to my mind: My God, forgive him, because I already forgave him. The truth is, I don't know why", she added thoughtfully. "I think I know why" I said. Although you didn't know, he was being tried in the heavenly court where his near future was being debated. Apparently, the argument that "the accuser" was using to get him convicted was all the evil he has done to you all these years. Probably, the Spirit of God moved your spirit to finally forgive him and that empowered "the defense" to win the case. One and a half months later, the offender left death behind and accepted the Lord, fulfilling the favorable verdict that he was given.

The Bible repeatedly shows us that our lives and actions are under constant legal scrutiny. Job chapter 1 is not the only irrefutable reference, there are also mentions of God's role as the Judge of all the earth, of Jesus Christ and the Holy Spirit as advocate and intercessor, of satan as the accuser, angels as bailiffs, demons as jailers, etc ..., and that is what I based myself on.

It does not matter if you believe that you are nobody or that nobody sees you, each of your actions (and decisions) causes a reaction in the spiritual world. But this is important to know, not only for those who act badly, but also for the offended, since although she could allege the damage that he did to deny him forgiveness and subsequent absolution, later in that same court, she too would be tried for lack of forgiveness.

God help us to act according to His justice always, remembering that there is an accuser who does not rest nor have mercy.

"Declare me innocent, oh God! Defend me against these people who live without You; rescue me from these unjust liars." Psalm 43: 1

Avoid adaptation disorders...

In the last few months I have basically heard three different complaints: 1 "It's incredible, they act like nothing will happen!" 2 "They do not protect themselves, they have a defiant attitude. They say that you have to die of something!" And, 3 "I think this has got the better of him and has made him a little (or very) crazy." They seem like three different attitudes, but no, they are three sides of the same coin: Reaction to stress.

Faced with a certain crisis, our experiences, beliefs, gender and received information, influence how we react to the problem. Our mind will always try to protect itself in first instance, even endangering our own physical integrity (or that of others). The person will deny that the enemy exists, will challenge him or flee directly and outrageously in order to protect themselves, as we are seeing now. We should not criticize, we should understand that fear makes them behave like this. As Christians who know God and His word, our behavior must be different.

We know that these world crises are predicted in the Bible, that the coming of Christ is near and that, in the meantime, our God is the One who protects us and holds our times in His hands. Take care, yes; but most of all, get closer to your Lord and obtain His peace; so that when the time comes to leave: He, our crown and an eternity of glory, will be waiting for us.

"These things I have spoken to you so that in me you may have peace. In the world you will have affliction; but be confident, I have conquered the world." John 16:33.

Containment measures...

The apostles felt the pressure after being imprisoned and receiving threats, so they met with the rest of the believers and told them what had happened.

The reaction was unanimous: "Let us pray!" *"Lord, the threats are evident, but we are not taken by surprise, since David, filled with the Holy Spirit, warned years ago: there will be opposition against God and his Christ "(Psalms 2: 1-2). So Grant your servants to confidently preach your word, and send your healing power so that many miracles and wonders may be performed in the name of your holy son, Jesus."* Acts 4: 23-30.

Nothing of what has happened has not been predicted. Perhaps different from that period, what currently threatens the spread of Christianity globally is a virus. However, God is still God, and He will respond to our requests for courage in preaching and for power to perform wonders and miracles of (yes, also) HEALING, in the name of Jesus.

Let us all come together and pray accordingly: courage to preach and power to heal; then let us act. God gave the power to His people to save the soul ... and also the body. He will back us up.

"When the believers finished praying, the place where

they were gathered shook. They were all filled with the Holy Spirit and they continued to boldly proclaim God's message" Acts 4:31.

The term quarantine refers to the process of undergoing isolation in order to avoid contact with any element that could endanger our security, for as long as it is considered necessary.

It is wise to always adopt self-caring behaviour but there are times when the situation requires extraordinary measures due to the ease of contagion or the severity of its effects. The reason for the measures in the current pandemic is obvious: but what about the possible collateral spiritual damage?

Due to the dangerous situation in which we are living, discouragement, anguish, and hopelessness can affect our lives and cause us to lose our trust in God. But is it so important to preserve our faith when what is obviously in danger is our body? Well, yes, because THE JUST BY HIS FAITH WILL LIVE; both in body and in soul and spirit and if we lose that faith, we can lose peace, joy (soul), communion with God (spirit) and even our life (body).

Protect your body, but also protect the rest of your being by isolating yourself from negative and discouraging words and feeding on God's promises.

"You keep in perfect peace those who always think of You and put their trust in You. Always trust in the Lord, because He is the eternal Rock" Isaiah 26: 3-4. (NIV)

Getting back to normal ...

"I do not know who has told you that you are finished, that God's plans in you have ended, that you have no remedy for your failure: that is why your strength and your faith have abandoned you." Long ago I heard this praise live in my church from a singer-songwriter: a pastor of Catalan origin. Who would have thought that years later I would listen to his wife through an audio with a prayer request for him? Please pray for Bernardo, I have been called by Intensive care and he is in a bad way, agonizing with the COVID19 infection. Please pray for him; a plea that was mixed, movingly, with a repeated command: "Stop what you are doing right now and pray for him."

It was the early days of the coronavirus, which presented zero hope of survival, and this woman, who had practically been declared a widow, responded to the tragedy with a call for spiritual warfare: Let us pray for him! Thank God her husband survived impending death against all the odds.

When we believe God, the goal of our crises is not loss, but rather, let us be blessed and He be glorified. So do not fear; let it not matter to you if they tell you that it is about to be lost or that it has already been lost ... cry out and have faith, because even what we give up for dead, we can recover in God.

"In God nothing is lost, do not cry with despair or give anything up for lost ... there is still hope" Bernardo de Sabadell.

"Jesus said to him: Have I not told you that if you believe, you will see the glory of God?" John 11:40 *(NIV)*

HOLISTIC TREATMENT

Broad spectrum therapy ...

As a doctor, there are two basic areas that I must cover in my continuous learning process: the problem-disease (what, how, when, in whom...) and the way to solve it (treatment). I cannot deny that my preferred area of training is treatment, that is, the resolution of what ails my patient, what has brought him to me, so that I can try to restore his health.

Within this section, the elements that I like the most are those that fulfill a double function: to diagnose and to treat. Yes, because when the eternal companion of any doctor, namely uncertainty (And this, what is it?) lays the weight of his hard hand on my shoulder and I can apply a technique or medication that not only clarifies the reason for the problem, but that also solves it for me at the same time, I feel double satisfaction; since 1, I solve the problem; and 2- I spend only half the time I would spend if I had to explore various options.

I love Adenosine (what type of tachycardia is this?). I love Flumazenil (and why this coma?) Among other treatments. However, what really fascinates me is prayer. Prayer not only reveals the origin of any illness (spiritual, physical, emotional...), it also detects it even before it begins to show symptoms.

Prayer gives a differential diagnosis, not between two or three diseases, but between all of them. The best thing for me as a doctor? It solves them all; and for you? You don't have to be a doctor to apply this treatment! Do you know or suspect that there is something that is not going well in your life, but you are not sure what it is? Apply: "the prayer to your Father who is in heaven" and that disease will be diagnosed and resolved.

"Then the king of Syria sent horses, chariots and a large troop to Dothan. They arrived at night and surrounded the city ... The servant said to Elisha: - What are we going to do now, my lord? Elisha said to him: "Do not be afraid. The army that fights for us is greater than the one that fights for them. Then Elisha prayed and said," LORD, open my servant's eyes so that he may see. The LORD opened the eyes of the young man and the servant saw that the mountain was full of chariots of fire and horses that surrounded Elisha." 2 Kings 6: 14-17

Specialist intervention ...

He waited there patiently like everyone else. It was a gathering of sick people who were vigilant. From the moment they realized that the angel came to move the waters (which took on a healing power), they all ran to the pool, for the first to arrive received the miracle of healing.

The blind heard the noise and ran head first into the crowd. The deaf did not hear, but saw and ran; the mute likewise. But that paralyzed man could only lose: not only could he not run but he was alone, he had no one to help him get to the pool in time. Thirty-eight years passed in this way.

That day, Someone who was observing him and was moved by his situation, approached him and asked: "Do you want to be healed?" I do not know whether it was good manners or irritation at the obviousness of the answer, the paralyzed man answered him: "Yes of course! But how? when because of my type of illness I cannot get to the pool in time and be healed, and I do not have anyone to help me either.

What this man did not know was that he was talking to

the One who had created his body, created the pool where the miracle occurred and even the angel who descended to move those waters. Jesus healed him.

Sickness was not God's desire when He created man. Disease came along when man was separated from his Creator, as well as other evils, but He, in His infinite mercy and love for humanity, provided us with wisdom and the means to alleviate disease. However, if the time comes that the pool and the work of the "angel" do not work, we should know that there is Someone who has the power to heal the impossible. Let us ask Him, who continues to have the power and love to give us a miracle.

"Death had me trapped; I was overcome by the fear of dying. I felt terrible anguish! Then I begged God to save my life. My God is just and compassionate; He is a tender and loving God who protects the defenseless. I had no one to defend myself, and He came to my aid. " Psalm 116: 3-6.

Surgical drainage: Little heart inn ...

I read a text which I found interesting about how evaluating myself from time to time is healthy for my spiritual life. God also evaluated himself: *"And God saw everything he had made, and behold, it was very good"*. Genesis 1:31 Therefore we must also do it: *"Thus says the Lord of hosts: Meditate on your ways."* Haggai 1: 7

What is the benefit? Correcting our walk, improving our deeds, preventing our heart from following those paths to which it leans ... avoiding our spiritual destruction. I say it with pity for myself; because no matter how much I see the glory of God in my life, there are times when I forget the danger I am in, and there are even times when it is not that I actively withdraw from the Lord, but that distractions and anxieties make me forget that I have an enemy who has put a price on my head, and who is very patiently and constantly seeking the loss of my soul.

I have hundreds of visible examples, as I know you have too; but today I want to mention the invisible ones, those in which you have to fight without any other human being as a witness. In these cases, the battlefield is the heart. Here you see yourself surrounded, trapped, and with no way out, because you cannot decide not to return to that church, no sympathetic brother or sister will take your demand and argue with your accusers. Here there is nowhere to flee to nor cloak to leave behind, because your temptation down to is yourself, and the enemy does not answer you, but speaks, since it is your own voice.

In these last few weeks, and due to various circumstances, I have felt: anger, resentment, jealousy, envy, bitterness, pain, I have felt betrayed, mocked, belittled ... And the interesting thing about this is that I have felt justified: I have not done anything, they have done it to me. They have not taken my friendship, good faith, effort, patience, fear of God into consideration... And those feelings have established themselves slowly, until suddenly I have felt drowned in those wounds that have filled my heart. They have arrived so stealthily and from so many sides that I have hardly noticed when they settled in. My hands are clean, God knows I have done no harm to anyone, and because of this I feel so justified that I even start to justify these feelings which have come to make a home in my wounded heart. But there is a problem.

The problem is that I run an inn called: "My little heart", which has a rather demanding tenant. He does not like living with anyone else, what is more, he threatens to leave if I keep letting that rabble enter this inn. So he has demanded that I take stock of the establishment to see where those rats that disturb the peace of the house have got into, after which I must irretrievably remove them.

He is just a tenant, I tell myself, and others will come along. But I realize that He is the only one who pays me, that is, He is the one who maintains the inn. It is clean, tidy, He keeps the place peaceful and happy, that is, it is not a good idea for me to lose Him. So I decide to submit the inn to an inspection. I locate the rats' burrows, I see where they have entered, the damage they have caused, what is more, I can already guess what they are going to cause. I am locating them one by one and identifying them. Those rats are small animals and they even seem defenseless, that is why there are people who adopt them as pets, but how wrong they are to think that they are like that! What is more, I am able to confirm this when I try to throw them out. After hours of intensive work, I realize that it is impossible, and I begin to remember that another of the benefits of my Tenant is His willingness to help me in times of crisis. I call to Him for help, and in a moment, he has cleared the inn of those horrible creatures. There are no more rats.

As children of God we are bombarded throughout our lives to make us welcome bad feelings into our hearts. The Lord cleanses us when He becomes the tenant of our particular "little heart inn"; But many of the situations to which we are subjected on a daily basis make us open doors again for them to enter and make their nests.

God asks us to evaluate ourselves periodically. We cannot prevent them from hurting us, from betraying us, but they do damage the inn. Letting them live there hardens, corrupts, embitters and may even make the divine Tenant decide to leave. *"Look carefully, lest anyone fail to reach the grace of God; that sprouting some root of bitterness, hinder you, and by it many are contaminated"* Hebrews 12:15.

Assess yourself and cleanse your heart. Keeping it clean is more important than your dignity, or being right. Having it clean can depend on your relationship with God, and even your salvation.

"Above all else, guard your heart; because from it life flows." Proverbs 4:23

Behavioral therapy ...

We are all susceptible to being abused ... but we are also susceptible to being the abuser. Self-discipline, therapies, etc ... can help control it, but they will not heal you; and this is because there are spiritual forces that move around us, which we do not see, that can make us assume behaviors and habits that go against what is good; against what God has established as agreeable in His sight, and correct for good coexistence among those who are His most important creation on earth: human beings.

Those forces have sought, since Adam and Eve, to make human beings challenge and disobey their Creator out of sheer jealousy and hatred. As Saint Paul said: *"I know that good does not dwell within me, that is, it does not reside in my human nature. There is in me the desire to do good, but I cannot carry it out. In fact, I do not do the right thing, the good that I want to do, but I do evil that I do not want to do "*. Romans 7: 18-19

There are people who like to be dominated by evil to do harm; but many others bear these bonds due to various circumstances, without wanting to. I repeat, let us pray for the captives, anyone can be one. Only God can deliver the abused ... and the abuser.

"That is terrible! Who will save me from this body that causes me death? God will save me! I thank Him through our Lord Jesus Christ." Romans 7: 24,25a

---

Universal free health ...

Many people think that Christians are people who feel perfect and that when they approach God it is because they are looking for a bubble where they can take shelter so as not to "contaminate themselves" with others, whom they consider impure.

Nothing is further from the truth. We convert to Jesus Christ because Christianity is for repentant sinners; for people who recognize that they are not good and that they need help to change and mercy to be forgiven; things that only our loving Creator can give.

God is available to all human beings, but unfortunately only those who recognize that they need him, those that cannot go alone, approach him. While we are on the crest of the wave (young, healthy, well-fed, surrounded by loved ones, etc ...) God is expendable but when the bad times come, we realize how small and bad we are and how much we need Him.

If you find yourself in "that" moment, remember that Jesus wants to get close to you, love you, forgive you ... don't be ashamed; He knows us, he knows that we are "dust".

"Jesus heard them and answered: "Those who need a doctor are the sick, not the healthy. And I came to invite sinners to return to God, not those who think they are good." Mark 2:17. (NIV)

The Healing of Tortuous Wounds

The couple were embracing tenderly. I adjusted my focus, since it was not difficult for me from a distance to realize who they were, and ... what a surprise! I was assuming it was a pair of newly-weds, but the couple who were watching the rest of the town at a party from that semi-hidden place were a married couple of at least 14 years.

Who could have thought it, when months ago her mother came to our little congregation asking for help? She mentioned a drastic change in her daughter after meeting someone through social networks. She decided to dissolve her once successful marriage with children to live the "new love" she had found.

The church got to work without taking into account that the girl was not a believer, nor that the mother was of another denomination. The congregation prayed fervently to the God who served them and who can do everything; believing in His will that families should be united and husbands be faithful and happy; so a battle plan was declared.

The prayers were intense. There were moments of discouragement, for example, when she threw her husband out of the house saying that there was no turning back; or when the neighbors mocked them by placing an ox's horn – which is a symbol of infidelity – at the entrance of the town. However, we did not lower our guard, we kept praying and my eyes saw the result: they got together again, with a pledge of love and forgiveness and an intensity in their eyes and in the way they treated each other that made them look like a couple of teenagers.

I say this because I have seen it. God is a specialist in solving lost causes, forgiving unforgivable sins, healing indelible wounds, in bringing back to life things that were already stinking because they had died so long ago.

If we want to change ourselves or our circumstances, let's turn to Him; only He can do it.

"I swept away your rebellions like a cloud, and your sins like fog. Return to me, because I have redeemed you" Isaiah 44:22

Therapeutic support ...

In those days, my lessons were aimed in only one direction: attacking my emotions.

They have been conveniently brought to the surface and then systematically attacked, thus convincing me that a robot's life is very attractive and worthy of imitation: they do not feel, they do not suffer, and therefore, they cannot be hurt.

"My goodness Father! I could serve you better if I could disregard these annoying feelings. I would make the right decisions; I would not be angry at those who harm me; I would carry out the works that you entrust to me no matter the circumstances. Everything would be better."

Those are my conclusions. But don´t you find that when you are going through a challenging situation, everyone speaks about it? If someone delivers a message to you, it speaks about it. If someone lends you a book, the same... everything. Therefore, you assume that, apart from having to go through all of it, you should also learn the lesson properly, because if you do not pass the exam or the test on a certain subject ... you will have to take it again.

One of the points that has caught my attention when listening or reading about emotions is that it is not God's will for you to get rid of them (so, what happens to my desire of becoming Robocop?). God gave us emotions so that we can relate to Him and to other human beings. It is not His will that I override my feelings. What He seeks is for us to keep them under control, with the help of his Holy Spirit.

Let's see, how do I explain this to you and to myself? Yes, myself, because I've asked myself lately: why does God allow me to be in places where the people around me don't like me and they don't make any effort to hide it either? What's more, they are happy to prove it so that I have no doubts. To that question, I add another: why can't I, in response, let them know that I don't like them either, because of their behavior towards me and others? However, God makes me go over and share with them more often than I would desire.

This was the explanation: "You must learn to live with your emotions, not only with the beautiful ones like tenderness, gratitude, love, etc. but also with those of anger, resentment, envy, etc. because they are always going to be there, in your life, until you depart to be with Me. What I want to teach you is that you should not let any of those feelings dominate you, neither the beautiful nor the ugly ones. Feelings should not cloud your vision when deciding what to do, nor should they make you avoid being where you should be or carrying out the purposes for which you have been called."

"What do you want to do, Lyly?" He continues, "Give up the blessing of being in that place just because some people (or all of them) are upset? After all the effort you have made to get there? Whenever you receive a blessing and the enemy wants to take it from you, he will know that he will not have to do very much, he just has to make you feel rejected or inadequate. Will you allow this to happen? And what about My power? Have you not seen examples of how I have made people, who criticized and thought badly of you, admit that they were wrong and, in some cases, I have even made them become your best colleagues and friends?"

"Yes, you are right" I replied. "So what do you want me to do?"

"HOLD ON!" He replies "keep going, be blessed, do what you have to do, act as you should act and do not let your emotions dominate you. When you feel overwhelmed by them, do not let yourself get carried away; do not yell, do not hit anyone; go somewhere where you can be alone, even if it is a bathroom, and ask the Holy Spirit for help. He will provide you with the self-control you need (yes, that is how spiritual fruits grow).

God is using that circumstance for me to learn. His will is that I grow, and I cannot do so if I break down at the slightest provocation, or if I stop myself from doing the right thing because I love someone or I'm grateful to them for something. So, continue to feel and... Hold on!

"Our suffering is light and temporary and is producing for us an eternal glory that is greater than anything we can imagine. We don't look for things that can be seen but for things that can't be seen. Things that can be seen are only temporary. But things that can't be seen last forever" 2 Corinthians 4: 17-18.

Psychotherapy

Among the emotional needs of every human being, there is the need to receive respect from those around us. When that feeling is absent, the person perceives that they instead receive the opposite treatment, such as rejection or contempt from the people who are part of their social circle.

When this happens, most people will do their best to earn the respect of those around them. Sometimes they will do it with good deeds or with gestures that exceed their resources, with the sole intention of gaining the admiration of others. However, on other occasions, they can go over the limits of what is correct.

There are many sad episodes in which children get involved in criminal acts in order to be accepted in a youth gang. Girls or boys get into immoral situations just to avoid seeming inadequate or boring. What about adults? They incur debts of millions; which neither the debtor nor even their descendants can settle, just to have the approval of other members of their society. All of these are different scenarios and actors with a single objective: to obtain respect.

We are all gripped by the need to receive it, to perceive that we inspire it in others. Sometimes, as I have said above, we make efforts that go beyond the limits of our strength to achieve, only to be hit by the harsh reality that we are looking for it in the wrong places and that, therefore, we will never obtain the sense of fulfillment we dream of. Our thirst for acceptance will never be quenched.

However, there is a solution to this deficiency. We should just start by asking ourselves: Where are we looking for respect? Who has the duty to provide us with that degree of acceptance and in which order?

What a nice girl Arleen is, how selfless, helpful, etc.! It's lovely to hear people say things like that about oneself, but why go out of my way to convince others that I am like that? Can any of them really see my heart and really be sure that I have no ulterior motive in performing the act that fills them with so much admiration? Have you never felt fake when someone acknowledges something that, actually, isn't so remarkable? Either because it was your duty, because it is your job, because it is a mandate from the Lord that, as a Christian, you must carry out or simply because God gave you a natural inclination when he created you. In any case it has not come from you, so if anything, Glory to God who gave you the gift of serving others.

Even so, if you know how fickle human beings are, one day someone praises you and another day, out of the blue, they ask for your head to be chopped off and thrown to the wild beasts, why strive for the prize of such ephemeral respect?

I think the solution is that we must strive to receive respect from God. I am not saying theological nonsense. I am not talking about the salvation that is only obtained by accepting and confessing Jesus Christ as the only Savior. No, I am talking about living in such a way that Jesus speaks well of you in front of his Father *"The one who is victorious will, like them, be dressed in white. I will never blot out the name of that person from the book of life, but will acknowledge their name before my Father and his angels"* (Revelation 3: 5). And may the Father remember you fondly, as He does with David in His holy word: *"After removing Saul, he made David their king. God testified concerning him: 'I HAVE FOUND DAVID son of Jesse, A MAN AFTER MY OWN HEART; he will do everything I want him to do"* (Acts 13:22). Or how he spoke of Job, Noah, etc.

God is not fickle, nor is He bipolar; therefore, let it be God who speaks well of you. It is a great prize, since he compels us to want to do things with the right intentions, because we cannot deceive Him. Before Him, we will maintain our value, no matter if today "I like you or tomorrow I don't like you". He does not make us to do things that are beyond our reach, since we start from the premise that we are accepted through His son Jesus Christ and that our Father knows our capacity. Therefore, he does not ask us for more than we can give.

Do you feel the need to be respected? You are not the only person who feels that way, we all need it, this is very true. However, it is much truer that you must start from the right premise, because if not, you will inevitably be disappointed and hurt, if you have not been already. I, at least, already have many scars.

My medical advice is to do things in such a way that you feel at peace with God. People will recognize you sooner or later ... and if they do not, it does not matter. It is God who must know the good things you did and He will reward you for them.

"Since you are precious and honored in my sight, and because I love you, I will give people in exchange for you, nations in exchange for your life" Isaiah 43: 4.

"Nothing in all creation is hidden from God's sight. Everything is uncovered and laid bare before the eyes of him to whom we must give account" Hebrews 4:13.

Self-pardon...

Due to problems with my refrigerator, I had to have breakfast at the health center where I work. Just something simple, a cheese sandwich, but when I put it on the stove it reacted as all cheese does: by melting, and it ended up on the burner.

I had no idea that burnt cheese smelled so bad and so strongly, affecting, not only the common area for employees, but also the surgeries and the administrative area. It made me feel bad, and I felt worse every time one of my co-workers came in and asked about the unpleasant smell that was permeating the health center; to which the others responded by pointing out the cause and the person responsible of such a stink-bomb.

As the minutes and people went by and while I was eating my cheese sandwich (sorry, but embarrassment does not take away my hunger) two paths opened up before me. The first one, which I have gone through many times: humiliation, feeling excessively clumsy for having created an unpleasant situation for those around me who, until that moment, were having a quiet morning. The second, one that God has been teaching me in recent years: self-pardon.

Of course nobody wants to be the black sheep in a group, cause embarrassment to their family or fart in the middle of a meeting (sorry, but this is a message for all situations). Everyone, absolutely everyone, wants to be the star that shines the most; the savior of a situation, the one who has the answers to questions. And if we do not stand out for something good, we at least do not want all eyes on us because of something bad.

This is not always possible. If you do not make mistakes, you simply do not exist. Moreover, all the components of our society, both on a large scale, such as, for example, a nation; or on a small scale, like a family or congregation, make mistakes. The duty of each member is to forgive his or her partner and move on together. That is how it should be; because that mistake you made once will be someone else's mistake tomorrow; and the right thing to do is to forgive each other so that, as I said before, we can continue walking together.

We are not always going to have a supportive response from others, but it must be clear to us: if it was not our intention to err, hurt or harm, as well as asking others for forgiveness, we must also forgive ourselves.

After apologizing and finishing my sandwich, I got up from the table; I shrugged my shoulders and decided to take the other path: self-pardon.

"Brethren, if a man be overtaken in any tresspass, you who are spiritual should restore him in the spirit of gentleness; looking to yourself, lest you too be tempted" Galatians 6: 1

Transplant...

It could be called a full-blown trauma. Yes, the trips of several days or vacations that Nacha, my sister in Christ and flat mate, goes on could really be called: trauma. She only travels so that, when she returns, I can receive her with a piece of bad news: one of her beloved plants has passed away.

On this occasion, it was the orchid which suffered the misfortune. I think she died of sadness. She could no longer hear that singing voice that would wake her up every morning, telling her how beautiful she was and special she considered her to be. She died slowly while her carer (me) helplessly witnessed the daily decline, that persistent agony that impassively ignored my modest efforts to keep her alive. Now there is only one dry root left in her pot. I did what I could while I still had hope. In my mind, I went over the list of remedies that were supposed to keep her alive, things that Nacha had been repeating throughout our five years of companionship. I tried to carry some of them out, but was unsuccessful. One of these remedies was changing the pot.

The lives of living beings are not static, they are constantly changing. An example of this is plants. Eventually, they need a new environment that can contain that change of state. Sometimes they grow and their roots or stems no longer fit in the pot that contains them, or their roots rot because there is not a good outlet for the water, or because in the pot there is some sort of infestation that harms the plant, etc. However, the remedy to all of this is to change the pot.

Sometimes, we have the same problem as plants do, we need to change the pot. Get out of that place where we cannot develop or where we no longer fit. There comes a time when a place or a situation is too small for us, it constricts us and does not allow us to progress. It is a place to which we are already accustomed and, therefore, we do not want to leave. However, we cannot avoid it, in order to develop we have to be transplanted. Or else, our life will fade away just as happened to the orchid (and to many other plants that I have tried to look after).

You may be feeling the call to move away, to seek other horizons. Perhaps you have not grown out of the place, it could be that the place has become smaller, making it impossible to drain out the bad things, things that are incorrect, and therefore, your roots are absorbing waste, sins that are at the center instead of receiving clean water, the nourishment you need to keep your soul alive.

However, there is also the danger of direct attacks, of having the continuous threat of another living being who hides under camouflage, just looking like any other innocent leaf, waiting to attack their victim. Then, we will see the importance of changing the pot, preventing any plague from entering our domain and hurting us.

Most of the time, being transplanted hurts. It involves being uprooted from what, until that moment, had been your space, leaving your land for a new one, losing contact with what had been your source of life. On some occasions, you even have to amputate parts of your branches, stem or roots to prevent the damage from spreading, so you can start over clean, healthy and without pests.

I did not transplant the orchid. I do not even know if that would have been good for her, or, if it was, where I should have transplanted her. I do not think the orchid knew either. However, contrary to the orchid situation, there is Someone who cares for us and who does know when we need to be transplanted. He has noticed that our roots have overgrown the pot, or that our leaves are withered; or that a pest is mercilessly attacking them. That divine sower (Matthew 13:3) knows the land where we will prosper (v.8), and that is why he sometimes makes the decision to move us. That is why it is advisable to let Him make the decision, because He is the one who best knows when and how we should leave our pot; and which is the best place for us to build strong roots and grow in a healthy way.

Do you feel the need to change where you are? He will guide you on how, when and where you should go. Does leaving make you sad? You have not realized this yet, but you need to be planted somewhere else. It is time to grow and /or protect yourself against the lurking dangers. Receive peace, He is not like me: He does know how to take care of his plants!

"The Lord had said to Abraham, 'Go from your country, your people and your father's household to the land I will show you'" Genesis 12: 1.

Recovery...

All of us, at some point in life, or at many, have lost something or have had something taken away from us. Everything can potentially be taken away, even life itself. The respect we deserve, relationships, material possessions, hope, etc. can not only be taken away from us (because of situations or because someone steals them) but also we ourselves can lose them through our actions and attitudes.

Losses are always sad, even more so when we have worked hard for something to be with us, or when we already consider something to be ours, whether it is valuable or not.

The Lord brings to my mind that classic film *"Gone with the Wind"*. Magnificent performances and spectacular period costumes to recreate a story that leaves me with a sour taste. Regardless of the characters' actions, the film is a chronology of one loss after another. Scarlet O'Hara's character loses her family, her social status, the love of her life, etc. due to circumstances that, we can say, have nothing to do with her: war, other people, etc. Later on, she continues to lose things: her husbands, her children, etc. but this time it is because of her actions and attitudes. One way or another she loses, she is left empty.

The life of a real human being lasts much longer than the many hours a movie lasts. Seeing it in this way, I think that the sour taste that the film left me with could also multiply, just as the losses multiply when comparing reality to fiction.

Does this seem like a sad beginning for a reflection? Well it is not. Unless you think that there is no hope to recover what you have lost, what has been stolen or taken from you. Today is a good day to remember that there is Someone who can give back to you whatever the wind took away. That the situation does not have to end with you dressed in mourning, embittered, crying and making oaths that the wind will also carry away.

There is Someone who restores your honor, your good name, Someone who can give you back that broken relationship, your health, your peace, your lost possessions. There is Someone who sees your situation and your heart, who knows whether you have acted honestly or not and can return what was wrongly taken from you.

Call out to Him; mourn your loss in His presence and, I assure you, that contrary to what happens in the film, the wind will not take anything away, but will bring things back.

If, on the other hand, you were to act like Scarlet in the second part of the film, if instead of having your things stolen you have neglected them and lost them, God is still your answer. *"If my people, who are called by my name, will humble themselves and pray and seek my face and turn from their wicked ways, then I will hear from heaven, and I will forgive their sin and will heal their land"* 2 Chronicles 7:14.

If we cry out to Him, He hears us. Our heavenly Father restores, returns, He is pleased to return what has gone with the wind; whether it has been stolen from us, or if we have lost it... for Him there is no difference.

"Whatever is has already been, and what will be has been before; and God will call the past to account" Ecclesiastes 3:15.

PREVENTION

Mediterranean diet...

Empty calories are those that we can find in different types of food, to greater or lesser extent, with the main characteristic of giving us a lot of energy but little or no nutrients.

Refined sugars are a good example. It is true that they are delicious but eating them on their own and abundantly, in the end, will bring us obesity and other related consequences, such as heart disease.

"What is seen was not made out of what was visible" (Hebrews 11: 3b); and taken to the spiritual world, the "easy" "empty" gains are also those that do not provide us with nutrients, but will only bring us problems in the long run: we will get fat without nourishing ourselves.

Blessings, just like food, are meant to make us grow; improve our vision and other senses. They are also meant to renew our strength and prepare us for what may come. That is their purpose. That is how your Creator organized it.

Therefore, when you want to ask God for something, you must also ask yourself: what else will that bring me, besides a moment of joy? Will I be a better person? Will I have more patience? Will my faith and trust in God increase? Or do I only want it because others have it or because I want to feel superior to others? Asking God for a dessert/request with empty calories from time to time is not bad. Sometimes He even gives it to you without having to ask for it. But it is best to base your diet (material and spiritual) on a healthy menu. Your life, in general, will thank you for it.

"When you ask, you do not receive, because you ask with wrong motives, that you may spend what you get on your pleasures" James 4: 3.

You can't take back what you have already given...

The gentleman was almost 90 years old and was senile. He did not recognize his children, nor did he know who or where he was. But for some reason, his praise made me recall the prophecy. Due to his mental state, one good day he was staring at me enraptured and said, with admiration, "Beautiful!"

Long ago, during my last year as vice-president of a national association of Christian youth, in an activity in Bani a colleague from the board said to me, on behalf of the Lord "I give you grace. I will remove your tears; you will no longer be despised. When you walk down the streets, they will call you beautiful. Without expecting it, people you don't know will stop you in the street and will praise you".

It is funny, but later, during that year, the prophecy was fulfilled several times. However, I came to remember the Divine prophecy precisely through the words of an old man who had lost his mind. I laughed, thanked God for his goodness and faithfulness, and carried on going.

Days later, the same old man, who had been admitted to the internal medicine ward, stared at me again and with the room full of people, including my co-workers, he said in a very loud voice, "She's so fat!" This triggered an indiscreet laughter from everyone around. I comforted myself by thinking that I could not pay attention to a patient who had lost his mind. This led me to another thought: if I decide to ignore his mockery, I should not believe his words from the other day either. However, the Spirit made me discard that idea: the first time, he did not act willfully; he was obeying an order from God. The second time, whether it was the devil or him... It did not count; I was only meant to receive the prior blessing from God.

I remembered that while listening to the young woman. She spoke to me with a little resentment and bitterness towards her father. She could not believe that he had betrayed and disappointed her like that. "Do you know who that is? My own father!" I did not tell her about the decrepit old man. I only pointed out that on many occasions, and for different reasons, people who have been a blessing in our lives, who should care for us or guide us, disappoint us, hurting our hearts and breaking our trust. So, what happens then? Should we forget all the good they have done for us? Should we overlook our memories of when they were a divine instrument that made us prosper, the mouth of the Lord that guided us?

Why do pastors fall, leaders sin or exemplary ladies falter? Even more simple: Why does my brother insult me, why doesn't the church recognize me and why is my mother unfair to me? I don't have an answer for every particular case. However, what I can tell you is that if you did go through it, it was to make you grow. So that you understand that in those first blessings, those people have only been an instrument. The primary source of all your blessing comes from God, it is Him who you must honor first and in Him you must continue to put your trust, because He will never fail you. They, like us, are human and therefore imperfect, so eventually they will fail. Not once... but a thousand times. *"But we have this treasure in jars of clay to show that this all-surpassing power is from God and not from us"* 2 Corinthians 4: 7.

Has someone been a blessing to you and then failed you? Do not leave the church, do not end the relationship, do not become his enemy. Maybe they have had a bad day or are having problems; pray for them. Be an instrument of God yourself, for His blessing. Do not let them take away what has been given you, because it was God who gave it to you.

"But blessed is the one who trusts in the Lord, whose confidence is in him. They will be like a tree planted by the water that sends out its roots by the stream. It does not fear when heat comes; its leaves are always green. It has no worries in a year of drought and never fails to bear fruit." Jeremiah 17: 7-8. (NIV)

MEDICAL FEES

To our level...

I remember my emotions very well, when I arrived in Spain a few years ago: the excitement of finding myself in a new place, the uncertainty of what my next steps would be... However, when I began my training in Murcia, the place where I was living, the next thing that occupied my mind was the concern about which hospital and health center I could join.

"The best hospital to specialize in family medicine, here in the region of Murcia, is M" that was the general opinion. "The best health center, and due to its location (in the center of the city) the most convenient one, is the LF; but they are both" everyone kept telling me "difficult to access". Only those who obtained the first places in the contest could enter.

I had obtained a modest 15th place, and of the rest of my 16 Dominican companions, only two were in a higher position than I was. In other words, the possibilities of us obtaining the 14 positions that were granted to first year family residents in that hospital every year, as well as the four positions offered by the health center, were tiny, if not impossible.

The day came when the teachers in charge of each hospital and its associated health centers gave their speeches. This way we could discuss the characteristics and advantages of each place. When it came to the representative of the hospital M., with a rather arrogant attitude (which I must admit, I have not seen him adopt again in these four years), he spoke of the hard work involved in night shifts at the hospital, in addition to other difficulties. I do not know if that day he had had some previous upset, but the truth is that God used that circumstance to discourage most of the 44 residents who had selected the teaching unit of Murcia from entering that hospital.

The first to select the coveted LF health center was number 4, who chose the only position that had the option of selecting a hospital different to the one attached to the health center. Then number 6 got in, a Dominican Christian, and then my modest 15th place got in. The fourth was missing, so I prayed for another Dominican Christian colleague, and to the astonishment of the coordinator and the girl herself, who was in the 22nd position, she entered to complete the table of "residents".

The Coordinator not only had to swallow his negative prognosis regarding the possibility of us entering, he also had to admit (he already knew about our faith in God) that God answers prayers. At the M. hospital, out of the 14 positions we, "the morenitos", occupied 10. Moreover, at the elitist LF health center, our heavenly Father gave three of the four positions to three of His daughters, to the astonishment and scandal (I will cover that in another reflection) of everyone within the world of family medicine in Murcia. The subsequent years, as had been the case until the year we entered, the first places continued choosing the health center and the hospital in which I was trained.

The world has its rules, so does life, and they can only be broken by Their creator and Master: our God. If for any reason, we do not meet a requirement or reach a certain level despite our efforts, we should not be discouraged, let us trust. The Lord will lower the objective to our level so that we can take it in our hands.

This leads me to the following point: despite the discouragement that was widespread amongst the rest of the aspiring residents, God made us want to enter the hospital, regardless of the bad image that was given to us at that time. If God allows there to be a problem in order for us to access something that we desired and had been asking God for, let us not run with the general opinion. Let us be clever and see God's hand working on our behalf, and lowering things to "our level".

"David said to the Philistine, 'You come against me with sword and spear and javelin, but I come against you in the name of the Lord Almighty, the God of the armies of Israel, whom you have defied. THIS DAY THE LORD WILL DELIVER YOU INTO MY HANDS, and I will strike you down and cut off your head. This very day I will give the carcasses of the Philistine army to the birds and the wild animals, and the whole world will know that there is a God in Israel'" 1 Samuel 17: 45-46.

Traveling doctor ...

"If there is a doctor on board, please report to seat /carriage X and contact the flight attendants of the plane /train"

I do not know if it was a coincidence, but for a while, I heard this message through the loudspeakers on all the trips I went on. I even heard it twice on the same journey. On one occasion, having been very calm in my seat, I noticed that when I got up I started having palpitations. I was pouring with sweat and felt a tightness in the center of my chest; I was short of breath and thought that I could fall to the ground. "It can't be, I'm having a panic attack!" "It's impossible" I reason, "I face things like this almost every day at work, I don't have to be afraid of not being able to confront the situation".

Calmness seemed to want to return to my body after this sane reasoning, but in my head, the panic attack stroke back in a brutal way: "Yes, but you're thousands of miles above the sea, alone. If there are complications, what are you going to do? Will you ask the plane to land? They never have medicines in these places, nor is there anyone who even knows how to handle a tensimometer (that is true, at least that is what the flight attendants told me, unless they were lying to me!) You, facing this problem on your own?" All of this in a few seconds, but I recognized my enemy and decided to go on a tactical retreat to the bathroom before going into battle. "Lord, look at this anxiety and fear, they are not mine. And if it isn't anxiety but, on the contrary, it is a heart attack (they have similar symptoms), I also give you my trust. You are the one who guides me and saves me in every situation. You are the one who gives me wisdom and works for the health of those patients. Take away the fear, take away that voice in my head and come with me, let it be nothing, and if it is something, keep them alive until we land". My heart rate went back to normal, and the peace (that God gives and that surpasses all understanding) came back to occupy my cardiac armchair.

Sometimes, I cannot help feeling stressed out in a situation, be it because it is very difficult or because I just did not expect it. What I can avoid is allowing it to neutralise or destroy me... and I do this by praying, by requesting our Father's help. He gives me peace, enlightens me in complex situations and (I strongly suspect) he solves these problems that I face.

"And the peace of God, which transcends all understanding, will guard your hearts and your minds in Christ Jesus" Philippians 4: 7.

Who said it first?

A few years ago, while entrusting my next night shift to the Lord, I reproached Him in the most respectful way possible, though with a small hint of bitterness (I could not help it), for allowing me to find a job precisely as an assistant in the emergency area.

Of course I thanked him because in that time of crisis, in which there were so many people out of work, including doctors (even more so in my legal situation) He had performed the great miracle of giving me a job. But I was still resentful for the fact that it was in an emergency room, instead of a quiet consultation in a health center, from eight in the morning to three in the afternoon.

"Father, you know how emergencies stress me out: working till sunrise, on bank holidays and other special occasions; together with the fear of something serious happening and not being able to solve it. I know that You are with me; but I don't like this and I told you a long time ago to give me work in whatever, except for this".

He, very kindly I must admit, allowed me to let loose and then brought something to my mind: "It is true, you let me know, but I had already told you first that this was My will". At that moment, I remembered the ministry I had received years ago, in which the Lord, after telling me that the man I had prayed would be my husband, for more than two years, was not for me, told me:

"I'll give you someone special. He will take care of you, he will be sweet to you, he will take you to dinner when you are working at night..."

The surprising thing about this case is that, at that moment, undertaking a specialization did not even cross my mind. I had finished my bachelor's degree and, as the Lord had refused to allow me to take the exam and ordered me to dedicate my time to work with youngsters, I had assumed that my career had been put to one side. But after that ministry, I began to suspect that His "NO!" was not definitive, but more like a "not yet". This was fulfilled three years later, when he brought me to Spain to do the medical specialization.

During my four years of training, the promise that I would be in a hospital doing emergency night shifts was fulfilled. But the prophecy of those culinary treats, which would be brought to me with affection by that "someone", was still pending. So, in the last months of my specialization, I keenly awaited the fulfillment of this promise.

May arrived, and with it, the end of my training as a specialist in family medicine... but nothing had happened. Then I became fearful. Why? Well, because I know He always keeps His promises, so this could only mean that my adventures in the Emergency Room were not over.

Indeed, that summer there was not a lot of work in health centers, and, oh surprise! They called everyone to do replacements during the summer holidays except for me. And, with the salvation of a month and a few days, the jobs I managed to get were in.... I do not even need to tell you.

I must admit, I felt very low for a few days. "But Father, why are you being so cruel to me? You make me do what I don't want, what I don't like. I know that you want to make a brave vessel out of this clay, filled with trust in You; but I told you LONG ago that: I don't like emergency rooms!" And then he spoke to me:

"Don't be silly (that's what I understood), if I open doors for you in that direction, it is because that is the path that will bring you blessings. Besides, you know that even if you are clumsy (which you are), I always help you, I teach you to do things right and I lift you up.

"This is what the Lord says— your Redeemer, the Holy One of Israel: 'I am the Lord your God, who teaches you what is best for you, who directs you in the way you should go" Isaiah 48:17.

"What do you prefer: safety alone, or risk full of My anointing, which is what brings you success? I want to bring out the best in you and I can only do it when you trust Me despite your fears. Lastly, do not say that you told me a long time ago you did not want to work in an emergency room. I had already told you before that you were going to work there".

From then on, my attitude changed. It was the Lord who gave me this job, so He will help me and I will do well. It is not self-delusion, when I talk about "awakening hidden talents" and say that I have none! No matter how deep I dig, I won't find them. But if He has given me this job, it is because He is going to hand me the tools to do my job excellently, without mistakes, without fear.

Because that is the other side of the coin: If God has led you towards that type of job/ministry it's because that is where He is going to use/bless you. In the same way: if the enemy has decided to install fear/displeasure in you so that you don't go down that path, it's because he knows that God has a powerful purpose for you in that area.

At that moment, I rebuked the spirit of fear in my life. I arrived at my night shift treading firmly, happy and at peace; I understood that my Lord had given me this territory and had anointed me for it, therefore, I was going to do a good job because He was with me. There, I will wait for my treats when they arrive. There, I will hear His voice saying: "See? I told you so".

"I will instruct you and teach you in the way you should go; I will counsel you with my loving eye on you" Psalm 32: 8.

Ask about the purpose...

That Saturday I had a night shift. After taking a bath, as I still had a few minutes to spare, I decided to lie down for a while and, when I closed my eyes, I saw it. He was leaning on a table; he had straight, short black hair, parted to one side. When I enter the room where he is, he lifts his intense blue eyes and looks at me. I open my eyes, startled, what does this mean? "Ah, this must be the appearance of my future husband", I said to myself mischievously. I picked up my things and went to the hospital.

Upon arriving to the office, I greeted all my colleagues, the incoming and the outcoming. Among them, I saw someone that I had never seen before sitting at the table with his head down. If it were a bet I would have won, because he was the same man from my vision. I took a deep breath, finished greeting everyone with a slightly shaky voice, which nobody noticed thanks to the noise of the change of shifts, and went to put on my uniform to start working.

He was a temporary worker who only came in on Saturdays as reinforcement and I was only allowed one Saturday a month. However, that month by mistake (?) they had given me three Saturdays. For that reason, we coincided many times and became good friends; although the memory of that vision and its possible meaning haunted me and did not allow me to approach him or speak to him with confidence.

One day: "The other colleagues have told me that you attend the Evangelist church", he told me. "Yes, that's right; what about you, are you religious?" "No, I'm an atheist and I don't believe in those things, there is no scientific evidence". "Ok" I said to myself, "then this is my purpose" I thought. I started preaching to him. We were interrupted by patients arriving, other colleagues' conversations... but as I saw that he kept looking for me to talk, I kept talking to him.

At a certain moment, when it had all turned into lecturing and justifying, I cried out to God and he brought me his *rhema*: "You talk about life being unfair; and that if there were a God, He would be to blame and man would be an innocent victim. But that is not it, we are living the consequences of our sins. Possibly, childhood friends of yours who had the same opportunities as you did have now been destroyed by vices. And yet you are a doctor: healthy, young and about to start a family (yes, he told me that he was engaged).

His eyes widened and for a moment he was a little sad and absent, as if he had remembered something... or someone. God, who looks inside our hearts, had put his finger on a sore spot. He listened to me meekly when I told him about the testimony of Juan Luis Guerra, whose songs he had listened to; and I played the song that says: "I don't need sleeping pills, if you're with me".

After preaching to him, we stopped bumping into each other. We did not share any more shifts. I heard that he got married and stopped doing shifts at the hospital soon after. But I know that he was brought here, and that I saw him in my vision, because God had a purpose. He did not convert at that moment, but the seed was there, ready to germinate at the right time.

"As the rain and the snow come down from heaven, and do not return to it without watering the earth and making it bud and flourish, so that it yields seed for the sower and bread for the eater, so is my word that goes out from my mouth: It will not return to me empty, but will accomplish what I desire and achieve the purpose for which I sent it" Isaiah 55: 10-11.

The enemy can sense God's purpose in a given situation; be it at the beginning of a friendship, a new job or a place we go to... and he will try to fill us with prejudice so that we do not fulfil what God wants us to do. It may not be the same prejudice he used with me, as a single woman; but he will find a way to make us feel shy, get distracted and lose the opportunity to fulfil the purpose. When we are faced with a situation that makes us doubt, let's ask the Lord about his intentions, and let's walk through them, fulfilling them.

God has made me laugh...

A few years ago, I asked the Lord which medical specialization I should take. I had almost finished my internship and, as a rule, as a matter of course, it was time to do the necessary paperwork in order to, possibly, enter a glamorous specialization such as neurosurgery. I, just as the rest of my colleagues, expected that someone who God had blessed with such good grades (God opens doors and makes you obtain good results, I can assure you of that), would select something prestigious, as well as profitable.

When I prayed to confirm what I had already assumed to be a fact (although I could say that I was seeking God's will), I got a surprise, because the answer-guide that I expected from the Lord was not about what to choose, but about "not choosing". Bewilderment, anxiety, tribulation... all of this came into my life. "What will I tell my parents? After graduating with honors, they expect me to be a cardiologist at the very least, so they can brag about it. My colleagues had entered or would enter specializations such as gynecology, urology or oncology. What was I going to tell them when they asked me? Most people: brothers, family and friends in general, would question my ability and maybe whisper behind my back that, due to my incompetence, I couldn't get a job at a hospital after having studied for seven years".

I did not presume anything, my fears were not overstated, I lived through all of that. I'm not going to say that I was a saint, I gave up many times. Thank God I am not white because I would have turned red with shame when someone mentioned, with all the good intention, that I was a doctor and I did not know what to say to those who asked me which hospital I was working in.

No, I was not a saint, nor a paragon of faith when I cried in the presence of God asking for that job that he had promised me. "Take away my affront", I begged him, just as Sarah, Rachel, or Anna would have done when they felt sterile and wanted to produce a child. I was no example, but God continued to be God and gave me strength and comfort during the four years I waited, encouraging me to wait for the promise that, in the end, he kept. Because He, apart from placing love in our hearts, is the one who helps us with what we do. He was true to me and, today (I just realized), years later, he has shown me why he kept me waiting.

Through a prophecy, he told me one night in a service in the city of San Cristóbal: "You are going to laugh when you see what I have prepared for you, and you will understand why it has been so difficult and such a long wait". Today I cannot do anything but laugh. In the end, I chose a position as a family and community doctor in the region of Murcia. Nothing glamorous, in appearance, but it is what He chose for me.

My life is in God's hands, He is in control, He leads the way. Today I am where I should be, in God's time, in the way He has chosen, and I know that I will keep laughing because He does not change, He continues to do wonders; it is what He does best.

"For you make me glad by your deeds, Lord; I sing for joy at what your hands have done" Psalm 92: 4.

It is not the same...

Being wise is not the same as having knowledge. It should go hand in hand, but this is not always the case. A good and practical example is that I, as a doctor, can have a lot of scientific knowledge; but if I do not know how to apply it to improve the health of my patients, then something important is missing.

Wisdom is the practical and effective application of acquired knowledge. God wants us to be wise. Moreover, God commands us to seek, ask, and yearn for wisdom in ALL spheres of our life. He even goes further, by showing us that there is a greater wisdom than earthly wisdom, which we should seek even if achieving it means making a greater effort. *"Fear of the Lord is the foundation of true knowledge, but fools despise wisdom and discipline"* (Proverbs 1: 7b) It sounds very mystical, but it is impressively practical.

If, as a doctor, I know several ways in which I can cure or improve a disease, but instead of using the most complicated and expensive treatment or solution on a patient (for my own benefit), I use the easiest and cheapest because I know and respect God, then I am a physician with efficient and practical wisdom. But, why wise? Because I solve the patient's problem and because I avoid having problems myself, knowing that HE-WHO-SEES-EVERYTHING is fair and will repay me with the same currency or an even higher one if I do not act correctly.

This is applicable to all spheres of life: Let us get wisdom. *"Get wisdom; develop good judgment. Do not forget my words or turn away from them. Do not turn your back on wisdom, for she will protect you. Love her, and she will guard you" "but fools despise wisdom and discipline"* Proverbs 4: 5-6; 1: 7b.

While there is life there is hope...

The address was not clear, so we decided to ring the first doorbell at hand. "Good morning, have you called for an ambulance?" My colleagues and I asked him.

"Unfortunately, it wasn't me" the woman replied, "there is another house just ahead with the same number, but with the letter B, it must be there". We could not help it, her answer made us curious, so we asked her to clarify: "I used to call you frequently, because of my parents' multiple illnesses. Now I cannot do it even if I wanted to, because neither of them are here, they have passed away." Her face filled with sadness and we left to fulfil our duty in silence, not knowing what to say to ease her pain.

It is true that life would be simpler if we did not have problems or commitments, but we forget that where there is life... there will be problems and commitments. "I have to take care of a sick relative: Thank you God because I am not alone and I am important to someone!" "I have developed varicose veins with my pregnancy: Thank you God because I have been able to conceive!" I see it every day, we do not find happiness in things "not being complicated", but in appreciating and being grateful for what we have "despite complications".

"Always be joyful. Never stop praying. Be thankful in all circumstances, for this is God's will for you who belong to Christ Jesus" 1 Thessalonians 5: 16-18.

Call the good doctors!

A colleague told me this anecdote during a night shift. He told me that when they arrived at a patient's house, they saw he was in very bad condition, so they decided to take him to the hospital. While they were getting him into the ambulance, the patient went into cardio-respiratory arrest, so the team proceeded to resuscitate him. Between chest compressions and ventilation techniques, they hear the patient's wife screaming and repeating to them: "Make a call so the good doctors come, don't let him die!"

The emergency service outside the hospital has various levels, and the one destined to vital emergencies, with enough equipment to provide life support until it arrives at the hospital, is the mobile emergency unit (EMU). I suppose this is who the lady was referring to when she shouted: "Call the good doctors!" In actual fact, the lady (and all of us if we were in a similar situation), was within her right to request the attention of those who are supposedly better trained to respond to such a critical situation. But we can't receive everything we want.

To put this into context: The first minutes of cardiac arrest are key to resuscitate a patient, and not only that, but also to give the patient in question a decent quality of life post-resuscitation, due to the amount of time his vital tissues may spend without oxygenation (brain, kidney, myocardium...). Resuscitation should begin, if possible, within the first four minutes of the cardiac arrest. For every minute that defibrillation is delayed, the chance of survival decreases by 7-10%. Ideally, all cardiac arrests should be attended by the UME ("the good doctors"). However, the time it takes to go from the nearest UME base to the town in question is approximately 30 minutes, assuming that they are not attending another emergency when they receive the call, that they are already inside the vehicle and that it is heading in the direction of the patient's location. The advantage that "good doctor's" training does not provide – as they are regrettably 30 minutes away — would be provided by the timely intervention of a doctor who supposedly has less knowledge in resuscitation (supposedly...) and fewer resources; but who nevertheless is nearer to the patient. If we see it like this, who is the "good doctor"?

Ideals are seldom linked to reality. Ideally, on a rainy day, we would have an umbrella with us, but that day the weather forecast was wrong or we didn't see the predictions, and we get drenched. At hand, we only have a plastic bag.

Ideally, we would have that elegant umbrella that we keep at home, but if we do not want to get soaked, instead of complaining, it is better to place ourselves in reality, see how that bag can be useful and cover ourselves with it.

We need to focus on the fact that our ultimate goal, our real objective, is to solve this situation in the best way possible; regardless of whether the means that are within our reach meet our expectations. Do not interfere with the effective solution that the Lord has given you just because you can't have the one you think is best. Remember: in the time that it may take the "good doctors" to arrive, the patient could die.

"But Moses protested again, 'What if they won't believe me or listen to me? What if they say, 'The Lord never appeared to you'?' Then the Lord asked him, 'What is that in your hand?' 'A shepherd's staff,' Moses replied. 'Throw it down on the ground,' the Lord told him. So Moses threw down the staff, and it turned into a snake! Moses jumped back. Then the Lord told him, 'Reach out and grab its tail.' So Moses reached out and grabbed it, and it turned back into a shepherd's staff in his hand. 'Perform this sign,' the Lord told him. 'Then they will believe that the Lord, the God of their ancestors—the God of Abraham, the God of Isaac, and the God of Jacob—really has appeared to you' Exodus 4: 1-5.

Now that...

"Mary P.G!" I heard the voice of one of the wardens who takes patients for their imaging studies. I started to walk faster when I recognised my patient's name, who the warden was pushing in a wheelchair. "Wait, where are you taking her?" "To have a head CT scan and X-rays on various parts of her body," the orderly replied while reading the application. "But that's impossible. Who asked you for those tests?" I asked.

I had gone to see her half an hour ago. Her consultation was about one of her frequent episodes of lumbosciatic pain, secondary effect of some very clear, studied and confirmed herniated discs. She was given an anti-inflammatory and, after checking her history and re-evaluating her case to confirm that it was just another of her usual crises, I had left her in the waiting room, waiting only for her symptoms to improve in order to discharge her.

I checked the medical record number that the warden had and saw that they were different. After a deeper investigation, we discovered that there were two patients with the same name in the hospital at that time. The other patient had been involved in a major traffic accident including head trauma, which was the reason why she was going to have a head tomography as well as everything else.

"Mrs Mary, you knew that we weren't going to carry out any image studies, why were you letting this man take you for X-ray scans" I kindly reproached her.

"Oh darling! As I'm already here, it doesn't hurt to have a few tests to check that everything is ok."

Thanks to my Christian education, I decided to guide this lost soul down the right track, gently instructing her on the dangers of frequent and large amounts of radiation, but she didn't believe it was that important. I also talked about public spending and the delicate economic situation of the public health system, a situation which, as I suspected and she confirmed, she didn't really care about either. As it was impossible to get my message through to her and I felt like I was about to lose my self-control, I made sure that the pain had improved and I discharged her.

I wrote this reflection on health a few years ago and I

cannot resist taking it to a spiritual level; after all, "what is seen has been made out of what cannot be seen". You see, avoiding the unnecessary use of resources is something of which we need to be aware. We should not carry burdens that God has not placed on us. There is a dose, a weight, a load that has been determined for our shoulders, calculated carefully so that we can carry it (God does not overload us...). However, sometimes, due to lack of understanding, things we misinterpret as solidarity or simply defiance; we assume problems, worries or debts of others. Then we blame God when things don't go well for us or when we realize that our whole life is a long series of problems. How could it be any other way? If we carry other people's problems as well as our own, and at the times when we should be resting or feeling blessed, we get busy trying to solve problems that are not ours.

Of course, we must help others, but everything has a limit, we must learn to say no. I cannot carry other people's burdens; I cannot stop feeding my family or stop paying my bills to cover for others, because we will both be left with nothing. God give us wisdom.

"And why worry about a speck in your friend's eye when you have a log in your own? How can you think of saying to your friend 'Let me help you get rid of that speck in your eye,' when you can't see past the log in your own eye?" Matthew 7: 3-4 (NIV)

Dissection

It was past two o'clock in the afternoon. We had already finished our day's work and, after making sure that there was nothing pending, my tutor and I always proceeded to carry out the second part of our work together: assessing my performance in the part of the consultation that I had carried out alone (always with a phone nearby for questions and calls for help). We would go over the daily list and comment patient by patient, until we got to a patient that inevitably made me put on an upset expression:

"I had a little disagreement with him."

"What happened?" enquired my tutor.

"Well, since he arrived he asked for you and when I informed him that I would be his doctor that day, he spoke to me in an off-hand manner. I tried to treat him in the kindest way possible, but he didn't care. That didn't really bother me, but he said he wanted a prescription for some antibiotics that he had bought at the pharmacy for a toothache, in order to pay for them"

"And what did you do?" asked my tutor. "I told him that if he didn't show me an indication from the dentist, or let me check his mouth to see the infection, I could not prescribe an antibiotic, it was unethical. The patient threatened to file a complaint and notify you and I told him to go ahead, because you were the one who had talked to me about an ethical and rational prescription". I concluded, reproducing slightly the adrenergic signs of tachycardia, tachypnea, etc. that the confrontation had produced in me.

After finishing my explanation I looked at my tutor; I noticed that he was trying to find the right words to answer me and I didn't like it. Whenever he agreed with my decisions, he responded quickly and enthusiastically. This reflective preamble, I suspected, meant that he wasn't going to agree with me.

"I agree that the correct thing to do when giving out a prescription is making sure it is backed by a professional opinion. However, there are times when we feel overwhelmed by the attitudes of a patient and, when we reach a point where we feel that we have control, the power to decide, we let them feel the weight of that power. You may have wanted to act ethically, but could your decision have also been affected by the desire to restate your authority, before someone who challenged it from the moment he entered?"

I felt like an onion, whose layers were being removed until it was completely exposed. In a second, and with a few words, my tutor's clinical eye dissected my intentions, and peering through the wound was the ugly face of my ego.

At that time I was a fourth year resident. I felt safer in clinical situations and in doctor/patient relations, even in those special situations where I had to convince a patient that: "I am qualified to treat you, even if you want Mr So-and-so to see you because 'He knows me and my medical history'". At least that's what I thought.

I realized that I still had to grow; and that also included evaluating my motivations when making a decision in a stressful situation. Furthermore, if I wanted to push the ugly face of my ego away from my medical decisions, I had use my power, it is true, not over my patients, but over my actions and myself.

*"Do not be quick to say who is right or wrong. Wait until the Lord comes. He will bring into the light the things that are hidden in men's hearts. He will show why men have done these things. Every man will receive from God the thanks he should have."*1 Corinthians 4: 5 (NIV)

Either my opinion or yours...

A few months ago, while on duty, I received a call from the emergency coordination service asking me to go to a house with my team in order to attend an unconscious man. After arriving at the scene and assessing the patient, it was clear that we were facing cardiac arrest. He was a man in his early 80s who had already had several heart issues. By the look of it, this was going to be the last trick his old heart would play, refusing to continue beating.

In general, in the case of an elderly patient admitted to hospital, with poor quality of life and little or no probability of being effectively resuscitated in the event of an arrest, the decision could be made with family members (and left in writing) not to attempt resuscitation if there were a cardiac arrest. However, this was a patient who, despite all of his characteristics, I did not know and I was in his house. I had a decision to make.

Therefore, in my initial evaluation, I not only paid attention to the patient's condition, but I also took the opportunity to intuitively assess the family members. There were many and they were weeping inconsolably. Their crying was not gentle and resigned, they were crying loudly, so I did not hesitate in my decision: we began to perform a heart massage, placed an oxygen mask around his mouth and electrodes in case he needed an electric discharge. As was expected, we only managed to get tired and break one of the patient's ribs, but he was already a corpse. There was nothing else to do.

Shortly afterwards, while I was having breakfast in a café, I went to pay but the waiter didn't allow me to. A woman, who identified herself as one of this patient's daughters, had already paid. She appreciated the interest and work dedicated to trying to save her father's life, although many of her relatives and neighbors thought that we had exaggerated. It was quite clear that he had died instantly; but still, she wanted to thank us for the effort.

A week later, another of the deceased man's daughters arrived at the health center, she was accompanying a friend. She told one of the nurses who had also assisted her father that she was upset with us because she felt that we hadn't done enough to save her father, and that was the reason he had died. The same situation, two points of view. Has anything similar ever happened to you or is any resemblance to reality pure coincidence?

Every decision we make in life will have people for and against it. If you listen to one side, the other will feel disappointed; and if you listen to the other, the first side will say that you are making a mistake. It is good to listen to advice, but if you are the one who must make the decision, because it is you who will bear the responsibility, I advise you not to base that decision on what others think you should do, but on what you think is the right thing to do.

Either of these opinions could have made me feel bad, but I was so certain that I had done the right thing that any other opinion was invalidated, regardless of whose it was.

Do you have a decision to make? Ask the Lord for direction to know what the right thing to do is and then proceed. Do not put the desire to please others before your peace of mind.

"The Lord makes firm the steps of the one who delights in him" Psalm 37:23.

Careless carer...

I was listening to the daughter while she was giving me a full report on the little improvement that she was experiencing, according to her mother, after the arthroscopy. I eventually laid eyes on her father, who was sitting next to her, and had a weird expression on his face. This expression could well be attributed to the weariness of having to care for a patient who demanded so much health and family care, as was the case of this lady. However, what most caught my attention was that his face never changed, despite his daughter having changed subjects from her mother's complaints to her parents need for medication.

"Excuse me for the interruption; has your father always had a crooked mouth?" I asked the daughter.

"Oh, I hadn't noticed, but I don't remember ever seeing him like this"

"Mr. José **, have you noticed that you have a crooked mouth? Since when has it been like that?" "It's been that way for a couple of weeks" He answered with an unclear voice.

"Does he always talk this way?" I turned to his daughter again, who was astonished and looked at her father intently, as if she wanted to make up for the little attention she had paid him in recent weeks.

"I hadn't noticed, doctor. The thing is that we are all so worried about my mother, including him, that we had not realized. Besides, as he has always been so quiet, we didn't realize he couldn't speak properly."

I checked with the person in charge of the shift. It was a neurological condition that had started developing a couple of weeks ago. We referred him in order to assess his possible admission as an outpatient to do a study or begin treatment. We requested everything that we considered appropriate, after informing the patient and his family that the diagnosis was probably a stroke with after-effects and telling them about the future steps they should take.

I wrote about this experience a few years ago, as an example. The figure of the carer is essential in any situation that requires someone to take care of others who, due to their age or specific needs, are in need of it. A mother or father, a sick person's carer, a social or spiritual leader... whoever is a carer is expected and/or required to do so with devotion and responsibility... but they also need care.

Abishai and the rest of David's army knew this, that is why in 2 Samuel 21: 15-17, we observe that, after seeing that the life of old King David was in danger, his leader/carer in the battle, Abishai, who was looking out for him, ran to defend him. Then, together with the other soldiers, he ordered him never to go out to battle again "so that the lamp of Israel will not be extinguished". In other words, they were taking care of their carer.

A carer is an invaluable asset to achieve personal, family or group goals. We need someone to be in charge and make decisions, or to channel those decisions in order to achieve success or stability, depending on what it is that they are taking care of. That is why the incidents that may surround this figure must be taken into account. A small child cannot take care of their father/mother, but those of us who surround them must make it easier for them. The elderly members of a family, a church, a community, etc. we must make life easier for those who are in charge, recognize them, honor them or help them from time to time. Criticize a carer if they achieve a goal but part of their flock is lost along the way; but criticize the flock if they achieve their goal at the expense of their carer's wellbeing.

"Have confidence in your leaders and submit to their authority, because they keep watch over you as those who must give an account. Do this so that their work will be a joy, not a burden, for that would be of no benefit to you" Hebrews 13:17.

An old enemy again...

While I was on duty, I received the call. A woman over

80 who had suffered a cerebral thrombosis just a few days ago suffered a new episode of loss of consciousness, so I had to go and see her.

Her family explained everything to me in a few minutes: the patient had spent the last three days with her eyes closed and made little or no response to her family's conversations. As she had been discharged a few days ago, they decided to wait to see if she recovered, but seeing that time passed and she was making no improvements they called the emergency coordination center to ask for a home visit.

"It's the same situation as before" one of them told me "I think it's another thrombosis", said another. I approached her, and after the nurse had checked her vital signs were adequate, I began to examine her. The woman was completely unaware of what surrounded her, her facial expression did not show any sign of suffering. Only her right arm, which had been affected by her recent stroke, was bent, but given her current state of consciousness I had no way of knowing if it had gotten worse. I proceeded to pinch her (or to assess if she was reacted to pain, which sounds more scientific) and noticed that she would withdraw, but she still didn't regain consciousness.

I already had enough evidence to confirm the opinion of the family members who filled the room (now that I think about it, why didn't I ask them to step out?). However, in the haze of making this fast resolution, the rush I was in, the family's approval of me supporting their opinion as a diagnosis, the hunger of not having been able to eat tea or dinner due to the number of patients I had treated, not to mention the ones who were still waiting for me at the center... I saw his face, the face of an old enemy of mine.

Show me the medication she is taking again, I told another relative (they were many, it seemed as if they were at her wake). They pulled out the list and there I saw the name written down: benzodiazepine. I looked at the patient and I saw it even clearer, there was no longer a mist "It's you", I said to myself. "Will you take her to the hospital, doctor?" another relative asked me. "Give me a moment" I replied, "first I must do something". "Load a flumazenil and inject her with half an ampule", I told the nurse, "There is something I want to confirm".

It was almost instantaneous, the mist totally dissipated after using the antidote and my old enemy revealed his face, allowing my patient to open her eyes widely and smile gently towards her relatives, as if waking up from a profound sleep, which in fact was the case. "It's not another thrombus", I told my surprised audience, "what happens is that they have given her too many sleeping pills".

Benzodiazepine poisoning in the elderly is a very common problem in Spain. It happens even when they are administered low doses, due to kidney function deterioration, respiratory problems, forgetfulness or other frequent pathologies in the elderly. This makes poisoning more frequent than we think and, sometimes, it can even be mistaken for other health problems.

I have fought this enemy several times. In my years of training, I spent hours treating and studying patients who we suspected had suffered brain accidents, respiratory insufficiencies, comas, etc. but, in the end, God would enlighten me and solve the problem after hours and procedures, suspecting there could be benzodiazepine poisoning and administering the patient with ampoules of its specific antidote: flumazenil.

This is how it happens in our lives. God allows us to face that personal enemy again and again (weaknesses, difficulties, limitations, insecurities). And, although at first we fall defeated and ashamed (repeatedly), there will come a time when, after having faced him on so many occasions, we will be able to recognize him even at a distance. No matter how he has disguised himself, no matter what others may think or what your feelings tell you; you know him so well, you have faced him so many times, that you can see him from afar and you defeat him. That is what we call: EXPERIENCE.

Are you in that phase of continuously falling even though you don't want to fail? Do not be discouraged, ask God for strength and keep getting up as many times as necessary. Because behind all of this there is a purpose: that you recognize your old enemy anywhere and you help others to defeat him just as you will have already done.

"Simon, Simon, Satan has asked to sift all of you as wheat. But I have prayed for you, Simon, that your faith may not fail. And when you have turned back, strengthen your brothers" Luke 22: 31-32. (NIV)

The Light Gospel

Despite my wishes, I lost the draw: I would have to work the second shift. With that in mind, I went to rest for a few hours, and when I returned to the observation area I found an unusual amount of movement. My colleague proceeded to give me a relief report of each patient before leaving, after which she warned me: "three of them are in a critical state"; and then she gave me some advice: "at the slightest problem call the assistant doctor to come down and help you, because they could die on you". I remembered the last time I was on duty with the same assistant. I had to call her due to two complicated patients and, the time it took her to come down (which may not have been long, but because of the situation I was in, seemed like ages), was the most agonizing moment of my entire experience doing night shifts at a hospital. I made a request to the Lord in my head: "Father, make sure I don't have to request any help, You are going to take care of me and guide me".

The other assistants from the first shift were also leaving and felt the need to give me the same warning: "Things are looking bad, if you see that you cannot control the situation tell the assistant to come down sooner". Instead of just evaluating the situation, I also evaluated myself and found that I was at peace telling God: "You are my assistant, and no one here is going to have complications". I proceeded to do my job and administrate the medication orders. The most complicated patient was also very agitated, despite the strong medication. He did not calm down and his condition wouldn't improve; then I realised it could be a good idea to give him a certain treatment. I checked that there were no contraindications, but in the end, I chickened out and didn't administrate it.

Time flew by and the assistant doctor in charge came down. I informed her of the condition of each patient and she decided to treat that patient for his restlessness. She prescribed various medications and, in the end, the patient managed to sleep precisely after having received the one that I had thought of. I reproached myself for not obeying the voice of my "Celestial Assistant" and I finished the watch in peace.

Light is an English word and it means "ligero" or "liviano" in Spanish. Something light is easy, stress-free, without difficulty; and God wants us to live such a gospel. We may stumble sometimes; face difficult situations, paths that we must inevitably go through… However, our attitude and the way we take these situations on may vary. We can feel that we carry all the weight of the world, that we have the worst luck or, on the contrary, we can think that the problem is easy, and that it will be solved because God is in charge. That is possible, that is to live a "Light" gospel.

The light gospel isn't something I want to sell you, it is not a "new gospel"; On the contrary, it is very old, it is the one that God stated in his Word: "In this world you will have trouble. But take heart! I have overcome the world." John 16:33. It is living without fear because you know that everything is in God's hands, including, above all, you. It's knowing that nothing takes Him by surprise, because He already knew from the beginning of time that this was going to happen, and that even if it happens, in the end, it will all turn around in your benefit.

I like to live the light gospel. That night I was at peace, instead of being scared and having an anxiety attack or an attack of hysteria, as I would have had before, for being alone at dawn with those patients who needed intensive care. I invite you to live the light gospel, I recommend it to you as a doctor; the peace it produces protects your heart, slows down the formation of wrinkles; avoids high blood pressure, gastric ulcers, hair loss; your nerves stay in control... Ultimately, it is good for physical and emotional health, and much better, for spiritual health.

"For my yoke is easy and my burden is light" Matthew 11:30. (NIV)

THIS DOCTOR HAS ALSO NEEDED HEALTHCARE

The Doctor's doctor...

My arrival to the country would be a surprise, I planned it that way. I waited for the service to end so that I could greet my aunt, who was sitting several rows ahead. However, something happened.

The pastor of the church was preaching on health, and in an act of faith, he asked the audience to place their hand over an aching part of their body and then ask God for healing. I did not hesitate. I placed my hand on my abdomen and prayed to the Lord for my intestines.

For months, I had suffered from painful discomfort, changes in my bowel movements and I also felt a bump on the right side of my abdomen. These were worrying symptoms for someone who knows about health. The prayer ended and I went to greet my aunt. After the initial surprise and hugs, she told me that she suspected that I would soon return to the country, because the night before she had dreamed that I was in a service where her pastor invited us to pray and I placed my hands on my abdomen. Would you say it was a coincidence? Not if you know God.

A year went by and after being struck by continuous doubts I decided to have a colonoscopy. Before, I prayed: "Lord, you told me that you had healed me, I believe You. I will go ahead with it and trust that there is nothing; and if there is, You will allow me to discover it in time to remove it (God ways are multiform). Result: a colonoscopy negative for malignancy.

If you know or suspect that a disease is knocking on your door, do not be overwhelmed or let anxiety you bring you down. First of all, present your case to the Lord. Even before making an appointment for that consultation or for those studies, put it in the hands of the One who can change diagnoses or heal diseases no matter how established they are.

"Cast all your anxiety on him because he cares for you" 1 Peter 5: 7.

Panic attack. Who said fear?

A social network suggests that you publish a memory; a few years have gone by. In the picture, I appear on my first night shift as a specialist assistant in a hospital emergency department. Several years later, with much more experience and better abilities, I continue to work in an emergency room; facing delicate situations such as cardio-respiratory arrest, intracranial hemorrhages, different types of shock, traffic accidents and even giving diagnoses for cases that are not always clear.

Sometimes I surprise myself. Not because of the situations that I face, but because it is I who am facing them. All my life and in all situations I remember being a fearful and apprehensive person; so much so, that my aims (anyone who has known me for years can corroborate this), could be reduced to finishing my degree and dedicating myself to teaching, which was familiar to me, at university. I wouldn not get near a patient in my life! The reason was that I did not feel capable of doing it properly, because fear came hand in hand with insecurity, as if it were not enough.

I finish my studies with honors, but I felt the Lord stopping me so I would not opt for a specialization. Without the prospect of continuing my training and with the literal terror of facing an emergency with a patient, I decided to work in an office. One day, I met an ex-colleague from university who warned me: "You cannot continue like this, medicine is a science you forget if you don't exercise it". She was right; the theory that I had learned would expire, because medicine is a changing science. Therefore, as time went by, I could be compared to any first year student in terms of knowledge.

If I had done my specialization at that time I would have continued to advance, perhaps I would have slightly overcome my fear of patients, although it would not really be important because my goal was to be a university professor. However, I didn't, because I dropped everything.

Time went by and I practically forgot what I had learned. What led me, in the end, to continue through this path? A promise from God. He told me that I had not chosen to be a doctor, but that He had chosen me for this profession. That I should obey him because he was going to bless me; but at that moment, I had to stop until further notice... and I did.

Four years went by and He spoke to me again. He brought me to Spain against all odds; he made me pass the exam and undertake a specialization. Sometime later, he gave me a Master's degree and a doctorate... More than I had ever imagined. However, His work has gone even further: he has removed fear and insecurity from my life. He did not work on the basis of my previous knowledge, which I had either forgotten or it was outdated; rather, he practically started from scratch.

It is clear to me, everything I have achieved I owe to Him. I'm not just talking about qualifications or skills, but also about conquering myself, my attitudes, rescuing me from my fears, putting an end to my palpitations, sweat and mental blockage. My achievements are due to Someone who has shown me that with Him I can do everything, since it is He who can and wants to strengthen me (Philippians 4:13). He is the one who has shown me what I could have easily overlooked, for He provides me with vision and wisdom.

"I will instruct you and teach you in the way you should go; I will counsel you with my loving eye on you" Psalm 32: 8.

Our greatest enemies are not always outside, but within ourselves. One of them is fear. Fear makes you discredit yourself ("I cannot, I'm not good enough, I have no worth…"), it nullifies you so that you can't move forward and achieve your goals. But let us be thankful and trustful, because our God has no limits. He gives you the victory whether you can or cannot; whether you are good at it or not; whether you are on time or your time has run out. God bless us.

"For the Spirit God gave us does not make us timid, but gives us power, love and self-discipline." 2 Timothy 1: 7.

Spiritual risk factors…

Despite the fact that some may have a physical or emotional origin, situations or conditions that we dislike can affect us spiritually.

Oppressive agents can enter through them, and they can also serve as gatekeepers that allow other oppressions in, to inhabit the house that is human life.

An ailment, someone dear saying something hurtful, a bad gesture, being mocked… can make us feel undervalued, rejected… and this, in turn, opens the door for the spirits of fear, rejection, self-pity, etc. Then, these oppressions will serve as gatekeepers for others, because they don't like to walk alone. Perhaps because I have the "middle daughter" syndrome or because of my parents' lack of expressiveness, I felt unloved. This brought eating disorders into my life, and after that, low self-esteem, fears, self-pity, anger, resentment, depression, envy, obesity, diabetes and a long etcetera.

It is true that, at the right time, the Lord gave me the freedom (even to make good decisions we need God to free our mind) of having stomach reduction surgery. However, being slimmer and physically healthier didn't involve a total liberation. To expel those perverse guests, one needs a power that no person or physical resource can give you; it is only possessed by the son of God.

Have you improved your appearance, demeanor, environment and still feel, or make others feel, miserable? Put your home/life in the hands of Jesus and ask Him to expel those nasty occupants. He is the only one who can liberate you entirely and forever.

"For he has rescued us from the dominion of darkness and brought us into the kingdom of the Son he loves, in whom we have redemption, the forgiveness of sins" Colossians 1: 13-14.

Riddle

I would always remember it and did not understand why. It mostly seemed like an unpleasant memory from my childhood and I did not think it had any repercussions on my adult life, until God gave me a revelation that day.

I was about 4 or 5 years old and I was behind the counter of a corner grocery store that belonged to my mother. My job was to keep an eye out in case a customer came in, after which I would call my mother so she could attend to them. Once, when there were no adults around, a man I didn't know came up to the counter and spoke to me:

"What a pretty, chubby little girl. Aha, you already have breasts! Turn around so I can see your bottom."

I crossed my arms tightly over my chest and, with my childish eyes, I looked at him with as much indignation I could gather. I cannot remember if I called my mother or if he just left; but since then, the memory of that unpleasant moment has come back to my mind repeatedly over the years.

"What an ugly old memory! Why must it always come to my mind? I was not hurt physically; he didn't put a finger on me (thank God). So, why do you bring back this memory, if he was just like any other creepy man?" I do not even know if he was actually a pervert or if he just wanted to pull my leg. The fact is that he didn't leave a mark on me... or so I thought.

Some time ago, I was reading about judgments that derive from the roots of bitterness and, according to what I understood: they are judgments, decrees or sentences that we establish against a person (it can be against ourselves) or situation, after living through an unpleasant situation.

After reading this, the memory came back to me. "Why does it appear now, why does this have anything to do with it?" Then the Lord reminded me of my attitude towards all the men who have approached me. How I have sometimes regretted losing the opportunity to start a new friendship, to meet someone interesting or to help someone who needs advice or a message, all because of my excessive caution, caused by the suspicion that whenever a member of the opposite sex approaches me he has bad intentions. Of course, in some cases I was right; But what about the others? Is it healthy to be haunted by this irrational and uncontrollable restlessness until I see that he isn't interested, until I feel safe?

Before that revelation, I would say that my attitude was because I was a serious and formal person, today I call it trauma. In words of the author of that article: judgments rooted in bitterness.

Due to that experience, all my relationships with the opposite sex were sentenced by the probability of them having an unhealthy interest when approaching me. For that reason, before continuing these relationships, I would inspect them to rule out any bad intentions.

Today, I want to be changed and live free. However, I have discovered something else, which is that I cannot do it alone. Just as I needed the help of the Holy Spirit to unravel that riddle from my past, I will also need it to: 1- Forgive that man for making me go through such an unpleasant experience which, although it occurred in my childhood, has cast a shadow on my present; 2- ask God to forgive me for my prejudices and wrong attitudes against all the men who approached me in an innocent way, without evil; And 3- to heal that wound in my soul, that crack in my heart, once and for all.

Today, I want the love of Christ, and not bitterness, to mediate in my relationships with others. I want my relationships with men to be determined by the premise that, whoever approaches me, is a creature of the Lord and that, probably, His creator has brought him to me because He has a purpose for him and He wants me to be his guide.

"See to it that no one falls short of the grace of God and that no bitter root grows up to cause trouble and defile many" Hebrews 12:15. (NIV)

Keep believing...

Everyone asked me the same thing: "Haven't you had a fever? Haven't you been prescribed antibiotics?" I kept answering: "No, thanks to God, everything has gone wonderfully. He has kept His word". However, there was a time when I allowed the resolution of continuing to believe to wear out. The devil realized this, due to the lack of security and firmness in my answers.

Yes, it is true that they did not vary much, but even so, the crack in my armor was noticeable; "Yes, I hope to God that everything goes well" "We'll see, God willing..." Then it happened, a suspicious liquid began to come out of the drainage I had on one side of my abdomen.

"Oh Lord! I told everyone what you said to me, that you were with me throughout the surgery, how come now there are complications? Where will there be a testimony?" One thing led to another: "If you never lie, then what is going on here?" I took a step back and looked at the equation again, then I realized that, in the first place, there was God's promise. Secondly, there was the miracle... But in the third place, instead of my faith, there were doubts. After seeing why the equation didn't add up, I decided to expel the interloper and reinstall my faith, which should be the sole occupant of that third place. Then, out of the blue, the suppuration went away just as quickly as it had appeared.

Do you know what was even more impressive? That it was exactly the same all through the first twenty days after the operation. Someone would give me a recommendation or tell me about their concern at the beginning of the day (with all the good intention, I am sure, but I am also sure about the bad intentions of my lifelong enemy), and, during the rest of the day, a handful of people would appear to offer me the same concern. Before long, I would begin to feel those miserable doubts lurking to regain the third place in my equation. Their intentions of making my blessing disappear would reflect on the symptoms I began to feel. However, moments later, the voice of my Lord would come to the rescue, alerting me to close the cracks and continue to enjoy my miracle. By obeying Him, the symptoms disappeared.

"Poor thing, it must be hard for you; you might have an

anxiety crisis because you'll no longer be able to eat what you like!" "Well, people who have that operation, if they don't take care of themselves, can get even fatter, up to twice as much!" "People with bariatric surgery usually end up vomiting and having other difficulties" "Now you will get a boyfriend and you'll leave the church". This was part of the bombing I received, disguised with a subtle veil of deceitful pity and sympathy. I must admit, they came close to evicting my faith from its clean and tidy third place.

A) The Lord promised me that He would make me lose weight. B) The Lord promised me that he would guide that operation and my recovery. C) The night before I was admitted, I fought a battle of liberation against the spirit of eating disorders that had afflicted me all those past years, and D) The way I recovered surprised everyone. However, I realised that the enemy never loses hope that he can spoil the party, because although it is a situation that affects the body, (though it can also affect the soul) it is a spiritual battle. I have received my promise, my miracle has been carried out, but if I want it to remain, if I want to continue enjoying it... I must keep believing, only then will I win.

"Arleen, how are you?" "Very good, thanks to God."

"Any pains?" "None, thanks to God."

"Some patients..." "No, not me. I am doing well and improving, thanks to the Lord." "No, I will not eat in the same way again. My stomach will not expand again. This operation will not be in vain. I will not become proud. My husband will fall in love with me because of my heart, not because I am thinner. I will not have a chronic deficiency of any nutrient. There were no mistakes made during my intervention, no! No! And No!... God will keep His promises!!"

Believe it, say it, post it. If the devil attacks you through doubt, resist him. He will have to flee from you and your territory.

"Submit yourselves, then, to God. Resist the devil, and he will flee from you." James. 4: 7. (NIV)

SELF-CONFIDENCE IN THE PRACTICE OF A PROFESSION.

Go get her!

"Doctor Arleen De León, please report to the nursing control room". I recognized the voice of one of my fellow residents. I raised my head from the report I was finishing off, I smiled at the patient in front of me and told him: "They're calling me, but don't worry, first I will finish with you".

I was not able to keep my promise because one of my superiors came over, she ordered me to stop what I was doing and report to the surgery room. Surgeons and radiologists were claiming my presence due to two patients with abdominal pain for whom I had requested, on one hand, a consultation for evaluation and, on the other, an ultrasound test. They asked me to justify these requests. I was calm and, upon arrival, I found the following situation:

Outside the cublicle I found both of the assistant doctors who were on duty and the surgery resident. Both their animosity and their intentions were clear: they were coming for me. They didn't believe that the two patients who I sent to their consultations at 12:30 p.m. had either a bowel obstruction or an acute abdomen. Therefore, they were determined to give me a class on physical examination, decision-making and treatment, and they acted as if they were Olympian gods: angry and condescending. They really made me feel intimidated! It was clear to me, and to those who were watching: if I had failed to diagnose any of them, my criteria and my honor as a doctor (despite supposedly being in training, which meant they should be less strict) would be strongly questioned that night. Just because I had dared to call them, and at that time!

I had no delusions about my abilities as a doctor... or as anything else. I lacked self-confidence and, in the face of these circumstances, I felt even less confident than usual; even though in my opinion they did meet the criteria. I imagined the humiliation I would go through and the bitter taste I would be left with at the end of the shift, despite the fact that any doctor can make a mistake, even more so when they are in training. So I cried out: "Father, don't let them shame me! Work in my favour and support my decision." I do not know if I am an expert in medicine, but if there is something I do know is, Who to turn to when I am in difficulties. Oh yes, I have a master's degree in that!

Regarding the first patient: 1- The 1st X-ray was clear 2- Despite having defecated, the symptoms continued 3- One of the surgeons knew the patient because it was not the first time he had this problem and, as if this were not enough, 4- He was the father of a doctor at the hospital (which he had not told me). The decision was made in a blink of an eye: Immediate admission.

As for the second patient, and despite my masterful presentation of the case, they persistently ignored me. They asked for things that I had just told them I had already done or were in process. Then they realised, after feeling it themselves, that they needed to open the patient's abdomen as soon as possible. Their suspicion: acute appendicitis. I did not need to display my skills of persuasion with the radiologist on duty: they themselves asked for an urgent ultrasound.

Do not think that I felt victorious. Nor that I am showing of my skills as a doctor, that is far from true. In reality, I recognize my limitations: I don't have a good memory, I am very insecure, I am not dedicated, nor am I very decisive, and I am not very brave when I face emergency situations (God help me to improve). By admitting this, I want to recognize the power of Christ in my life: How he responds to our cries, not only protecting us or providing us with wisdom in our daily tasks;

but also, agreeing with us when we face dilemmas.

I have seen patients go from not having a fever to a 40-degree temperature in an instant, right under my nose, and under the noses of those who were questioning my diagnostic suspicion. Just so the Lord could support my work. To Him the glory. Am I a good doctor? No, I have an excellent God! Blessings from above.

"I begged the Lord three times to take it away from me. But he told me: "My kindness is all you need. My power is strongest when you are weak." So I will brag even more about my weaknesses in order that Christ's power will live in me. Therefore, I accept weakness, mistreatment, hardship, persecution, and difficulties suffered for Christ. It's clear that when I'm weak, I'm strong." 2 Corinthians 12: 8-10.

CONCLUSION OF THE DEAL

Our life is a gift we must take care of because, one day, we will have to render account to the One who gave it to us and explain how we have administrated it.

Taking care of our health is a duty, but doing exercise and feeding our body is not all that is required. As well as physical life, there is a life that transcends matter and the time we live on this earth, which also needs us to exercise and feed it in order to sustain and strengthen it.

Accepting Jesus will give us eternal life. However, after accepting Him, we need to keep listening to God through His word, speaking to Him in prayer and trusting Him. These actions will keep us spiritually strong, healthy and well fed.

It is true that food and exercise can help you slightly in this life, but there is another one beyond. Receive it by accepting Jesus as your savior. Do you already have it? Start taking care of it. God give us wisdom.

"For physical training is of some value, but godliness has value for all things, holding promise for both the present life and the life to come. This is a trustworthy saying that deserves full acceptance" 1 Timothy 4: 8-9.

ABOUT THE AUTHOR

Doctor by vocation, christian by conviction, writer by calling and leader by responsibility, Dr. Arleen De León Robert works as an emergency doctor in primary care in Spain, her adopted homeland since 2009. Through her social media blog, "Educando a Lyly", she shares her experiences as a believer with the aim of being a channel for holistic health, on behalf of the physician of physicians: Jesus, who not only seeks that we be healed and healthy on a physical level, but also in our souls and spirits.